Begin Where They Are!

An ACTIVITY BOOK to develop and improve VISUAL SKILLS through directed movement for YOUNG CHILDREN and individuals with AUTISM and/or DEVELOPMENTAL DELAYS

by Kathy Nurek, B.S.
& Donna Wendelburg, M.S., COVTT

Illustrated by Kathleen Patterson

Copyright © 2010 Optometric Extension Program Foundation, Inc.

The OEP Foundation, founded in 1928, is an international non-profit organization dedicated to continuing education and research for the advancement of human progress through education in behavioral vision care.

OEP Foundation, Inc.
1921 E. Carnegie Ave., Suite 3-L
Santa Ana, CA 92705
www.oepf.org

Managing editor: Sally Marshall Corngold
Cover design: Kathleen Patterson

ISBN 978-0-929780-28-3

****

Optometry is the health care profession specifically licensed by state law to prescribe lenses, optical devices and procedures to improve human vision. Optometry has advanced vision therapy as a unique treatment modality for the development and remediation of the visual process. Effective vision therapy requires extensive understanding of:
- the effects of lenses (including prisms, filters and occluders)
- the variety of responses to the changes produced by lenses
- the various physiological aspects of the visual process
- the pervasive nature of the visual process in human behavior

As a consequence, effective vision therapy requires the supervision, direction and active involvement of the optometrist.

****

Table of Contents

PREFACE	v
BEFORE YOU BEGIN	1
AN IMPORTANT DIFFERENCE	3
NECESSARY TERMS TO LEARN FOR SCHOOL SUCCESS	5
BODY ORIENTATION/BODY CONTROL	7
MYTHS TO THINK ABOUT	8
WATCH YOUR LANGUAGE	9
REMEMBER . . .	10
MOVEMENT	**11**
Balance	12
Standing	14
Stand and Bend at the Waist	15
Walk	15
Jump	16
Long Jumps	16
Jump Up and Down One Step	16
Jump Moving Target	16
Hop	16
Gallop	17
Skating on Paper	17
Skip	18
Add Trampoline or Rebounder	18
START/STOP	**19**
Ride on an Adult's Shoulders	19
Start/Stop for Other Activities	20
Start/Stop Advanced	20
Walking Rail	21
Add Rhythm on Walking Rail	23
Add Throwing and Catching with Bean Bags on Walking Rail	23
Balance Board	23
Stilts	24
JUDGE DISTANCE	**25**
BODY IMAGE	**26**
EYE FOOT and EYE HAND COORDINATION	**28**
Dowel	29
Add Balance	29
Eye-Hand with a Friend	30
Roll Balls	30
Roll on the Table	30
OTHER EYE-HAND COORDINATION TASKS	**31**
BEAN BAGS	**32**
Body Awareness	32
Drop the Bean Bag	32
Throw and Catch	33
Throw A Bean Bag at a Stationary Target	33
How Far Away???	34
Throw and Move	34
Throw and Clap or Slap	35
Dot to Dot, Bean Bag to Bean Bag	35
Breathing	35
Bean Bag On Your Head Trick	35
BALLOON ACTIVITIES	**36**
Hanging Balloon	36
Eye-Foot Coordination	36
Eye-Hand Coordination	37

BALLOON ACTIVITIES (Cont'd)

Add Rhythm	37
Add Balance with the Balance Board	38
Add Balance with the Walking Rail	38
Moving Target & Moving Individual - Trampoline	39
Free Floating Balloon	39
Add Balance with the Balance Board	39
Add Math	39
Add Singing	40
Balloon Volleyball or Tennis	40
Balloon Volleyball on the Trampoline	41
Other Balloon Games	41
Soap Bubbles	41

DRIBBLING   42

Increase Difficulty by Moving and Dribbling	42
Dribble to Music	43
Add Balance	43
Add Thinking	43

PRE-WRITING ACTIVITIES   44

Sticking Hands	44
On-Off Sticking	45
Sticking - Pen to Pen	45
On-Off Sticking with Pens	45
Scribble	46

VISUAL MOTOR ACTIVITY STATION   46

Sticking	46
Off-On Sticking	47
Jumping	47
Tracing	47
Draw on Back	47

HINTS FOR DESK OR TABLE ACTIVITIES   48

CHALKBOARD ACTIVITIES   49

Scribbling	49
Straight Line Drawing	49
Two Hands Drawing Two Horizontal Lines	49
Multiple Horizontal Lines	50
Multiple Vertical Lines	50
Continuous Vertical Lines	51
One Vertical Line, One Horizontal Line	51
A Circle	51
Two Circles	52
A Square	52
Two Squares	52
A Triangle	52
Dots	53
Connecting Forms	53
Roadrunner	53
Racetrack	53

TEACHING RESPONSIBILITY   54
PRINT SIZE   56
OBSERVE BEHAVIORS FOR SIGNS OF STRESS   57
RELAXATION   58
APPENDICES

Appendix -A- Pre-Reading	59
Appendix -B- Motor Skills	60
Appendix -C- Children's Vision and The Learning Process (Glossary)	63

REFERENCES   65

Preface

Patients with Autism Spectrum Disorder (ASD) often have severe, persistent symptoms due to problems in visual system function. As more individuals have been diagnosed with ASD, optometrists have been challenged to assess and treat vision problems in this population. This is not always an easy task.

When I began to provide vision therapy for patients with Autism Spectrum Disorder (ASD), I often found few traditional vision therapy activities that were right for my patients, particularly those with severe language and motor planning challenges. I read many, many books and articles on vision in individuals with ASD, yet found little on the nuts and bolts of how to modify specific therapy procedures and vision therapy programs for these patients. Browsing an overlooked shelf in our clinic, I found this gem of a book, *Begin Where They Are!*. I began to use this book both to develop activities for vision therapy sessions as well as to educate parents on home vision therapy reinforcement. Regrettably, the book was out of print and I could not order additional copies. Fortunately, the Optometric Extension Program (OEP) has again identified and filled a need by reprinting this book and offering it to OEP Clinical Associates as a resource.

Written by two vision therapists, *Begin Where They Are!* is a readable, well-organized activity book that provides information for providing vision therapy to patients with ASD and other developmental disabilities regardless of their starting point. Though brief and written in simple language, this book provides a wealth of procedures and ideas for variations to enhance many areas including body awareness, bilateral integration, laterality, vision-vestibular integration, visual auditory integration, vision-proprioceptive integration, general movement, visual spatial processing, visual gross motor integration, and visual-fine motor integration. A sequence of pre-writing activities is provided to prepare the patient for school writing demands.

Begin Where They Are! also describes core concepts of developmental vision in basic, easy-to-understand language including the difference between vision and eyesight, myths of vision, and the role of observation and objective testing in the assessment of minimally verbal patients with ASD and developmental delays. Drawing on their background in vision therapy as well as education and social work, the authors, Kathy Nurek and Donna Wendleburg, have thoughtfully included a section, "Watch Your Language" on appropriate instruction sets and language to support patients' efforts. In a section on "Comfort", the authors explain how behavioral signs exhibited by a patient such as wiggling, turning away, or echolalia should not be interpreted as poor attention or cooperation, but may be linked to a patient's stress, boredom or reaction to an inappropriate activity selection. Sections on "Teaching Responsibility" and "Making Choices" provide specific recommendations for promoting independence and generalization of progress in therapy to home and school.

I am delighted to see this book back in print. I hope that it continues to provide optometrists, vision therapists, parents, and others who work with these patients with valuable information for a long, long time.

Rachel A. "Stacey" Coulter, OD, FAAO, FCOVD
Diplomate, Binocular Vision, Perception, and Pediatric Optometry
Nova Southeastern University
July 2010

"Young children learn through the development of patterns - perceptual, behavioral, conceptual and combinations thereof. For the child who is lost in space there are no patterns. The mass of stimuli constantly bombard him/her with incomplete and inaccurate information. These stimuli lack order, sequence and prior experiential guidelines. Despite normal intelligence levels, learning is difficult or even impossible for the child with perceptual handicaps.

The senses of the child - particularly the visual and auditory senses - are amenable to learning (training) as an ongoing process in the life of the individual. These senses, or perceptual systems, can be exposed to the therapeutic intervention at a very early age.

"We can help the 'Lost in Space Child' find out who he is, where he is, and what he is."

Howard Coleman M.Ed., O.D.

Before You Begin

This book is for professionals and parents.

We encourage you to:
- Stimulate all aspects of the child's life.
- Celebrate each small step in the development of the whole person.
- Know that visual development is directly affected by motor development.

Work through success:
- Work from easy activities to harder activities.
- Work from short periods to longer periods.

Customize activities to match the individual:
- If you choose an activity that is too easy, skip steps.
- If you choose an activity that is too hard, go easier.

Jump:
- Jump from one section to another.
- Skip pages if you wish.

There is no right or wrong:
- Success will vary.
- The amount of time available will vary.

Before You Begin...

Believe

All individuals can learn.
Learning begins with movement.

How to get started

Important ingredients:

1. Begin where the child is successful.
    - If Adam can kick a large ball effortlessly, the next step is to use a smaller ball.
    - If Sue can catch one scarf with ease three times, the next level is one scarf five times in a row.
    - If Mary can work at a puzzle for 20 seconds effortlessly, the next goal is 25 seconds.

2. Change the activity.
    - If the activity is too easy, increase the demand.
    - If the activity is too hard, lessen the demand to make the task successful.

3. Have fun.

4. Change activities before frustration builds (regardless of who is frustrated).
    - Example: "Balloons aren't fun today. Lets work with balance."

5. Join in with laughter, cheer leading, humming and singing.

6. Celebrate success with friends and family.

Major Concern

This workbook gives concrete ways to help a young child or an individual with autism and/or developmental delays:

1. Become more aware of
    a. His/her body.
    b. His/her body in relationship to the world.
2. Become visually directed.
3. Become more independent.

Our goal is the development of the whole individual. Our emphasis is on developing the visual system as the leading sense organ. This workbook is designed as a guide in developing that system.

Developmentally, the eyes learn skills through movement. ". . . 80 % of learning comes through the eyes. . ."[1]

> "By the time a child is two years old, one can observe that the child's eyes are beginning to lead his actions. Vision, the sense with the longest reach, the only sense that can scan, is starting to take over as the primary tool of perception."[1]

By seven years of age the body should be lead by the visual system. "When a child reaches his seventh or eighth birthday, his concept of space should be well developed. Both sides of his body should be able to use his vision instead of his hands to evaluate space."[2]

An Important Difference

The importance of the ability to make meaning of what one sees.

VISION: The ability to react and interact with one's surroundings thus gathering and storing information.

EYESIGHT: The ability to see a certain size target at a certain distance (20/20).

Example: You can SEE this 中 clearly.

But can you make meaning out of it?

The goal of the Visual System:
An individual who can:

- see clearly
- follow exactly
- shift from point to point
- have stamina (can work for longer periods)
- coordinate with the rest of the body
- lead the body by age 7 1/2
- take meaning from what they see
- gather information from what they see
- remember what they see

Individuals with autism often:

- have poor eye contact
- look through objects rather than look at them
- use side vision rather than central vision
- sweep the room with the eyes rather than look at specific items

How does one visually evaluate a patient with autism, with developmental delays, or a young child?

When getting a visual evaluation from a professional, the answers to ordinary questions are often not easily attained from this population.

Should these questions be asked?

- Do you see double?
- Do you see blur?
- Do you have difficulty seeing at distance or near?
- Which is clearer, 1 or 2?
- Read the chart.
- Are your eyes bothering you?
- Are you having problems with your eyes?

Then, what should be observed?

The visual professional with understanding and experience with autism, developmental delay or young children will not expect to glean complete information about the functioning of the visual system through instruments or questions asked of the patient. An excellent history of the child from the parents knowing what the child does at age level or chooses not to do. Observing the child as he/she interacts with:
- The environment
- Familiar people
- Strangers

The professional may choose to use the Denver Developmental or other developmental scales to assess skills. It is important that auditory/speech skills are included since they are of major concern with individuals with autism. Recent school evaluations can be of help.

How does one develop a visual system?

Dr. G. N. Getman emphasized the motor system is critical for weaving the fabric of future vision development. When the motor system is compromised, vision perception is compromised.[3]

Body awareness and control of self must be developed before awareness and control of one's environment can be successful.

Let us begin at the beginning. Start with any directed meaningful movement initiated by the therapist and then add a visual component.

The child's world starts with his/her body, so we begin with body awareness through movement.

Necessary Terms to Learn for School Success

Laterality/Directionality

Laterality is the knowledge that my body has a top, bottom, sides without naming those body parts (top, bottom, left, right). Babies can be observed looking at their hands and you can almost hear them identifying, "Wow, look what I found! Two of them! They taste great, hold stuff and can move in all different ways!" Later the infant finds the feet. BECOMING AWARE OF is laterality.

Directionality is naming. Not only does the child know he/she has two arms, now they get names, right and left. This right and left naming can be confusing. Piaget identified the stages of directionality. Generally by 5 the individual knows that right arm and leg are on the same side. By six, the individual correctly knows right from left on themselves and by seven can project that into space. This means they can identify right and left on another person in any position and on the printed page (b,d,p,q,6,9).

Why Is Understanding Laterality And Directionality Critical For Academic Success?

Piaget explains that top and right (arm on the right side) need to be easily recognized before an individual will automatically recognize (P - circle on top/right of line). Reading and writing are goals for all individuals. These differences (b,d,p,q,6,9), are small directional differences (top, bottom, left, right). Understanding top, bottom, left and right on my body is necessary before an individual will recognize top, bottom, left and right differences in printed material. Will a directionality delay PREVENT me from reading? No! But it will surely slow you down. I, personally, had a directionality problem until the age of 30. I could read and write. But imagine having to stop and think each time you come to b,d,p,q,6,9, rather than knowing the shape automatically. Slow does not make reading and writing easy or fun!

Rachel And Linda Or Richard And Larry

To many individuals with autism, right and left have no meaning. So we name the sides, Richard and Larry (Richard and right start with R while Larry and left begin with L). Any names that begin with R or L could be used. Later it would be Richard your right leg and still later it would be your right leg. For boys, boy names are used. For girls, girl names are used. More effective is using a family member's or friend's name, as long as it begins with "R" or "L".

The following directional terms can be learned by moving body parts in directions mentioned. Next, place objects in that position.

Up	Down	Forward	Backward
Sideways	Beside	Inside	Outside
Behind	To the rear	In front of	Between
Close	Away	Near	Far
Above	Below	Over	Under
Top	Bottom	High	Low
Middle	Center		

Example: Top

"Sit on top of a stool."

"Place a bean bag on top of the stool."

Questions to Ask:

- Can you lean to the left?
- Can you lean to the right?
- Can you wave your left hand?
- Can you raise your left foot?
- Can you touch your left ear?
- Can you bend your right knee?
- Can you point to your right?
- Can you point to your left?
- Can you point in front of you?
- Can you point in back of you?
- Can you jump up?
- Can you bend down?
- Can you put your arms out?
- Can you turn yours toes in?
- Can you take one step forward?
- Can you take two steps backward?

Special Instructions:

- Stand near the table.
- Stand far away from the chair.
- The child is instructed to point to a certain place and then to move there.
    Example: "Point to the wall that is nearest to you; walk to that wall."
- Identify the location of various objects in the room.
- Ask the patient to:
    Move sideways across the room.
    Move close to me and then move away from me.
    Move from the front of the room to the rear of the room going over one object and under another object.

Body Orientation/Body Control

Body Orientation

Individuals with autism move through space but do not gather information that pushes development forward. Rather, they amble through space without space imprinting their senses or learning. Kelly Dorfman, MS, LD,LN, Past-President of Developmental Delay Registry, wrote that, "developmental problems are not illnesses caused by germs or a specific brain malfunction, but are a group of symptoms created when the body has been stressed beyond endurance." She calls it **"THE TOTAL LOAD THEORY"**. There is too much stress from too many areas to allow the child to learn through movement.

Body Awareness/Body Control

WHY IS THIS IMPORTANT? My body is home base. Understanding how to make my body work and how to control my body is critical. Teaching body awareness/body control is step number one for toilet training. Knowing when you need to move toward the bathroom means you have BODY AWARENESS. Waiting until you get to the bathroom is BODY CONTROL. An example at a higher developmental level is that you will find that as the individual learns body awareness/body control, he/she will be more aware of the areas around his/her body and will keep those areas more organized. We have many examples of individuals who kept a messy desk at school and a messy room at home until the body awareness and body control were well established. As body awareness/body control become automatic, both the desk at school and the room at home are organized with greater ease.

WHEN YOU FIND AN ACTIVITY ISN'T WORKING, GO BACK TO WORKING WITH THE BODY! Go back to home base!

Myths to Think About

Sometimes the biggest obstacles to success are messages that have been embedded into our minds, but which are, in fact, not true. Below are some common misconceptions:

- Not doing an activity always indicates unwillingness to cooperate.
- The sized print you use is determined by your age.
- The appropriate school program is determined by your height.
- Attention span is determined by your I.Q.
- 20/20 means the eyes are working perfectly.
- Not needing glasses means your eyes work perfectly.
- Short attention span means you need medication.
- An I.Q. test truly measures ability.
- Any person can pay attention IF THEY REALLY TRY.
- All people can learn to read in the same way.
- One teaching method can work for all.
- All people can learn in a group setting.
- Doing a task one time means you can always do the task.
- You must love to read. There are a lot of books in your house.
- Stamina remains the same.
- If you can read quickly and accurately for one minute, you can read quickly and accurately for 30 minutes.
- If you can read quickly and accurately in the morning for 20 minutes, you can read quickly and accurately in the evening for 20 minutes.
- Looking at someone means you are paying attention.
- Looking at someone means you hear what they say.
- Looking at something means you will remember it.
- Looking at something means you see and/or understand it.
- Carrots will improve your vision.

Watch Your Language

The helper's words set the tone for success or frustration.

SAY	DON'T SAY
Let's do this together.	Try harder!!
You've earned the right to have a harder job.	You can do better.
You did that so quickly and accurately. This tells me you are thinking and working.	You're old enough to do that alone.
Tell me if you need help.	No video games until you get that done.
We'll come back to that in a few minutes.	You're lazy
Let's take a break.	I can't stand you!
Let's clean this up.	You're careless.
How else could you do this?	No! Don't do it that way.
You got the first part perfectly!!	Can't you do anything right?
Would you like some help?	I'll do it, you're too slow.
Are your hands doing their job?	Get your hands off that vase!
What did you hear me say?	You didn't do what I told you to do!
Tell me about the picture you made.	That doesn't look like a horse.
What else could you add to your picture?	Finish the picture.

Remember...

Remember, to develop a whole individual takes time. It should be done in small steps with fun and love as necessary elements. The entire body must be involved.

Some weeks you'll have less time to work than other weeks. There are activities in the book that will work for you, others you'll skip altogether. That's just the way life is!

Keep changing activities and creating new activities, as you strive to stimulate the growth of the unique individual in your life. Rediscover the joy of exploring life, one wondrous step at a time.

Celebrate!

Celebrate always. Small gains lead to large gains. Set small goals. Find success daily. Create victory lists to share with others.

Tanya's I Can List

Smile
Walk
Make People Happy

_____
_____
_____
_____

MY VICTORY LIST

Read the list often.

Add to the list!

Movement

From Arnold Gesell: "A child is born with a pair of eyes, but not with a visual world. He must build that world himself, and it is his private creation..."[7]

The eyes learn to see as the body learns to walk and to move.

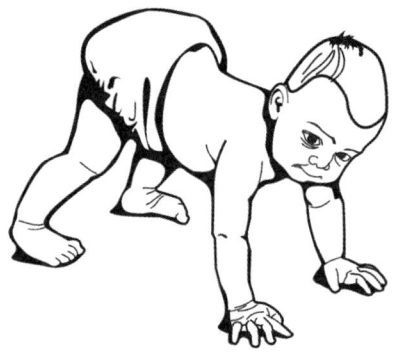

Keep in mind that children must crawl before they walk; they must pass through each of the motor milestones if their skills are to develop.[1]

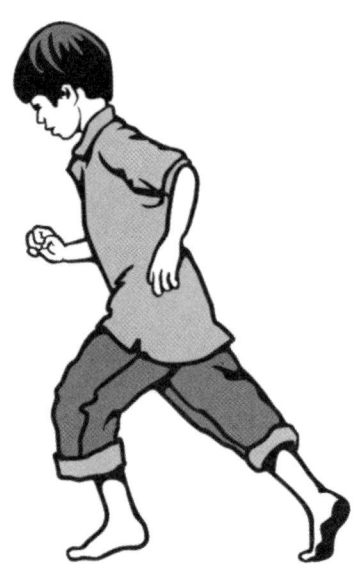

Movement can be seen as a basic aspect of development in children.[4]

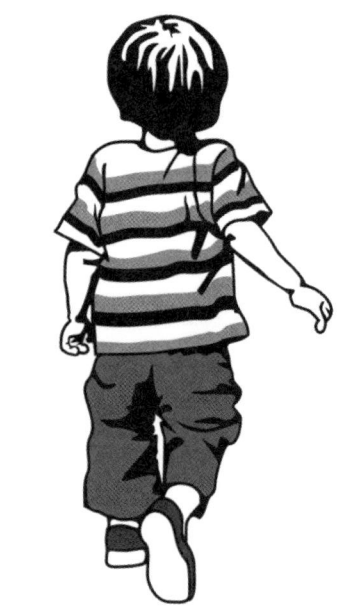

- Movement is essential for visual development.
- Vision is developed.
- Developed abilities can be improved.[5]

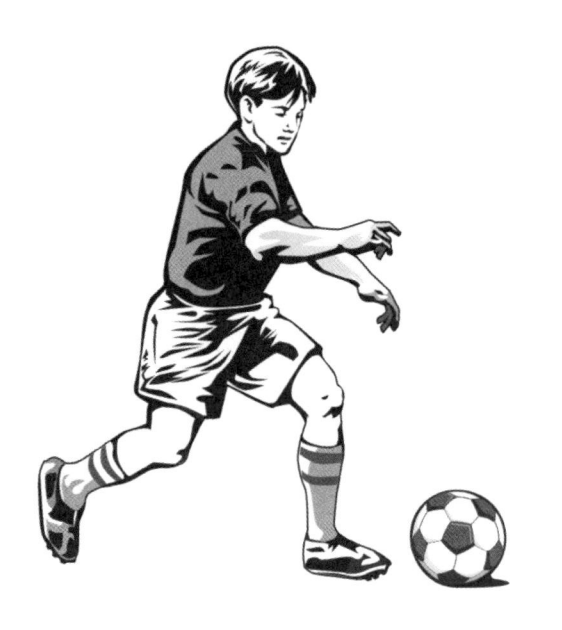

All behavior is movement of one kind or another. The movements made in a developing child constitute learning units that contribute to his total store of knowledge. Having developed awareness of his own body and having learned to control and integrate its parts, the child then goes on to build up a picture of the world around him.[6]

Angels In The Snow with Variations

Procedure: The therapist will move the body parts of the child until the child can move the body parts by himself. When the child can move the body parts, the therapist will touch and name the body part to be moved. "Jaclyn will move her Rachel-arm out and back." Later, the child completes the task alone.

Lie on the Stomach or Back

Glide body parts slowly on the floor.

    a. Arms and legs

    b. Arms alone

    c. Legs alone

    d. Right arm and leg.

    e. Left arm and leg.

    f. Right arm - left leg

    g. Left arm - right leg

Add:

    a. Answer questions (i.e. What is your name?)

    b. Rhythm

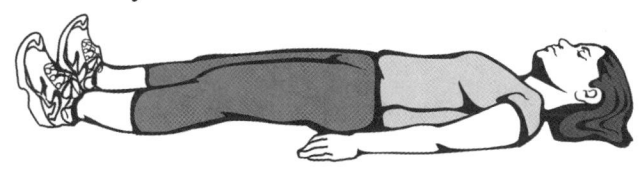

Lie on the Back

Repeat above movements while:

    a. Following a hanging ball with the eyes

    b. Talking (i.e. Tell a story)

Lie on the Stomach

1. Do swim strokes
2. Move like a snake
3. Move like a fish
4. Move like a caterpillar
5. Go in circles

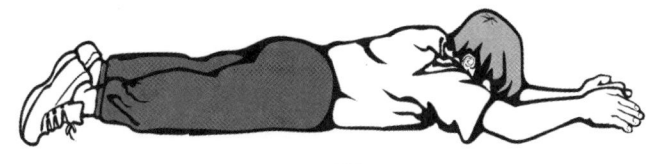

Hand and Knee position

1. Hands flat

    - fingers together

    - fingers point straight

Move:

    a. Left knee - drag toes

    b. Both arms at the same time

    c. Both legs at the same time (rabbit hop)

Add Balance

    d. Right arm with right leg

    e. Left arm with left leg

    f. Right arm with left leg

    g. Left arm with right leg.

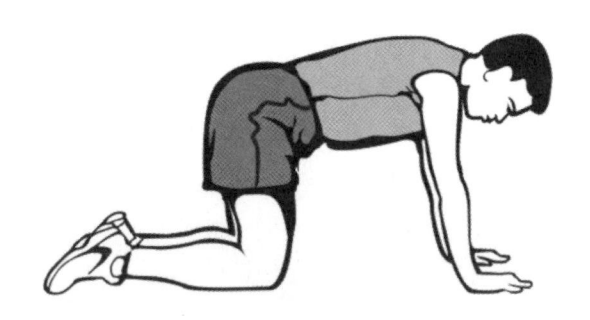

2. Eyes open, other times closed
3. Move the whole body as directed in relationship to an object (table, chair, box):
   a. Under
   b. Around
   c. Between
   d. In
   e. Circle
   f. Square
   g. Over
   h. Out
4. Lifting movements:
   a. Lift right arm and hold high
   b. Lift left arm and hold high
   c. Right leg - high and straight
   d. Left leg - high and straight
   e. Right arm and right leg out, up
   f. Left arm and left leg out, up
   g. Right arm and left leg out, up
   h. Left arm and right leg out, up

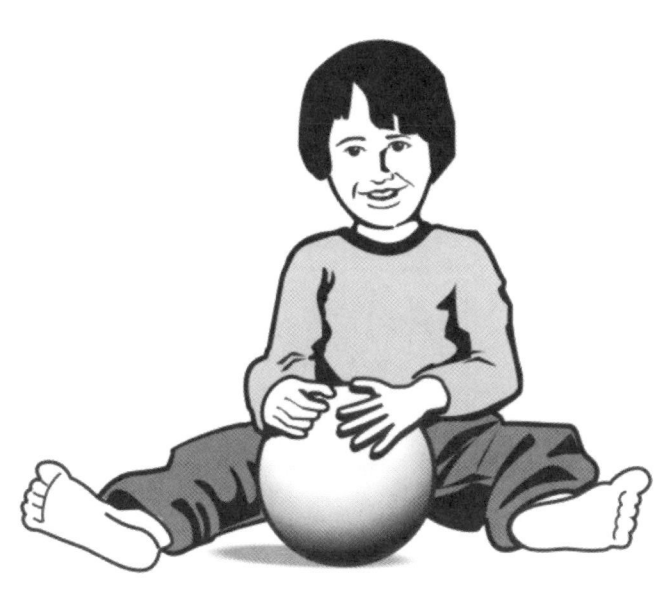

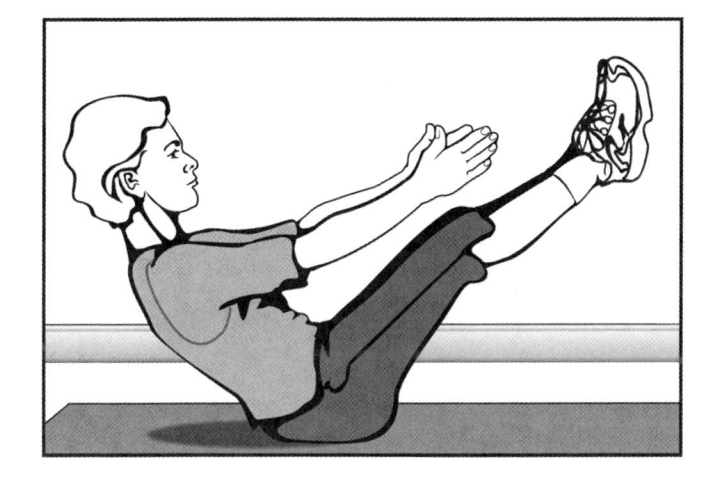

Sit - Balance on Buttocks
1. Lift arm and legs while maintaining balance.
2. Twist yourself around
   a. Use both hands
   b. Use one hand
   c. Use the other hand
3. Feet apart - together
4. Make circles with arms - legs
5. Arms go up - down
   a. Apart - together
   b. Right - left
   c. Near - far

Add balloon or ball
1. Sit and kick with feet
   - Balloon rolled to you
   - Right, left foot
2. Sit and hit with hand
   - Balloon or 9" ball
   - Right, left, both hands
   - Add balloon or ball
1. Sit and kick with feet
   - Balloon rolled to you

13

More Balance Activities

Purpose: To develop the two sides of the body as a unit. Balance of the body helps to develop a balanced visual system. Good balance improves safety. Developed balance allows one to move faster, turn corners quickly and show greater stamina. Athletes continually work on balance to maintain "the edge," as do seniors to prevent falls.

Standing

The proper standing posture is to have the feet the same distance apart as the shoulders.

Keep the feet stationary.

1. Move arms up and down
   - Say up and down (repeat)
   - As in jumping jacks
   - Straight up and down

2. Move both arms to the right and left (Rachel or Linda)
   - Say right and left (Richard or Larry)
   - Extend overhead
   - At waist
   - Swinging from sides

3. Circles
   - Large circles that cross in front of the body
   - Small circles
   - Eye height, shoulder height, waist height

Add Scarves

With a scarf in each hand, repeat the arm movements while standing.

Add Rhythm

Add rhythm and repeat the arm movements while standing. Chant or create a song using the name of the child and talk about what he/she is doing, "Ty is moving his arms in a circle. Around and around go Ty's arms."

Move in any pattern with rhythm.

Stand and Bend at the Waist

1. Right, Left (Richard or Larry)
   Say and bend (right - left)
   a. Body alone.
   b. Body and arms extended overhead.

2. Forward, backward
   Say and bend
   a. Body alone.
   b. Body and arms extended overhead.

3. Move in a circle from the waist
   a. Body.
   b. Body and arms extended overhead.

4. While on tip toes.

5. Bend knees and go low.

6. Change your feet position. Repeat the above movement patterns:
   a. On tip toes.
   b. With one foot in front of the other foot.

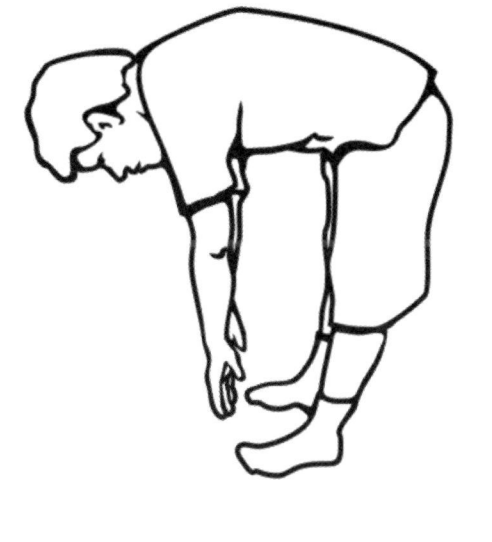

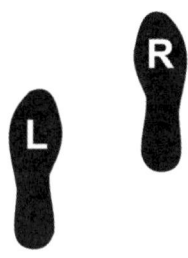

Walk

1. With arms at the side, walk forward and backward:
   a. at a fast pace
   b. at a slow pace
   c. taking big steps
   d. taking little steps
   e. raising knees up like you are marching
   f. on your heels, lifting toes up
   g. with toes point in or out
   h. as if you were on an incline (leaning forward or back like you were walking uphill or downhill)

2. Incorporate arm movements:
   a. Swing arms up when walking - right arm forward with left leg; left arm forward with right leg
   b. Swing arms across in front of the body

3. Create new steps
   a. Side step.
   b. Cross over steps.

4. Make up patterns
   a. Take 2 big steps and 1 little step (repeat).
   b. Take 3 fast steps and 3 slow steps (repeat).

Remember that both the child and therapist can create new patterns.
Any slight change in patterns should be applauded.

Jump

Equipment: string, rope, hula hoop, box, tires, or ladder

Arrange object(s) on the ground to create an obstacle course (i.e., using a string to form a circle). Beginning with the simplest object, instruct the child to jump:

- On	- Forward	- In	- Behind
- Backward	- Out	- Around	- In Circles
- Beside	- Left	- Right	- Between

1. Hold both hands of the child while jumping.
2. The child jumps alone.
3. The child jumps many times in succession.
4. The child first looks at the object, then jumps with eyes closed.
5. Repeat steps 1-4 using more challenging items that require jumping higher each time.
6. The child jumps objects in succession until he/she is able to jump all the objects.

Long Jumps

Create a ditch (with chalk, tape, string, rope) narrow enough to jump over successfully. Make the ditch wider with each success.

Jump Down and Up One Step

Both feet leave and touch the floor at the same time to jump down and up one stair step.

Jump Moving Target

Have several people standing in a circle with one person in the middle holding a rope.

Swing the rope in a circle close to the floor.

As the rope comes to each person they jump over it.

Hop

1. Hop in a circle pattern to the right.
2. Hop in a circle pattern to the left.
3. Hop on one foot to a particular rhythm.
4. Hop with that rhythm on the other foot.
5. Hop from one foot to another using a pattern.
6. Hop in and out of taped circles or a hula hoop.
7. With eyes closed, repeat 1 - 5.

Gallop

Move in a forward direction with the same foot always in front. One foot leads and then switch the feet.

1. Around a circle.

2. In different directions.

3. Pretend to be a horse.

4. To music.

Skating On Paper

Have each foot on a piece of paper. Keeping the paper under each foot, push the feet and the paper in a skating motion to:

1. Move around the room.

2. Do an obstacle course.

3. Have a relay race.

4. Go in circles.

5. Create a square.

6. Slide with; partner side-by-side or facing.

7. Slide forward, backward, sideways.

ADD:

1. Juggling.

2. Dribbling.

3. Thinking.

4. Multitasking. (Moving, juggling or dribbling and thinking)

Remember: Do activities for short periods of time, then longer.

Skip

If skipping is hard for the child, take his/her hand and go through the steps slowly. Say and do together:

"Rachel (right), step and hop"

"Lisa (left), step and hop."

Do the same thing when beginning backward skip.

Skip:

1. Around the room.

2. To music.

3. With a partner.

4. Through an obstacle course.

5. Slow.

6. Fast, maintaining pattern.

7. Forward and backward.

Add Mini Trampoline or Rebounder

1. Jump

2. Jump in foot patterns
   a. apart - together
   b. 2 hops on right foot;
      1 hop on the left foot

3. Jump in foot patterns while:
   a. hitting a balloon
   b. catching and throwing
   c. juggling

4. Jump and juggle while singing

5. Jump and sing

6. Jump and count, spell or do math

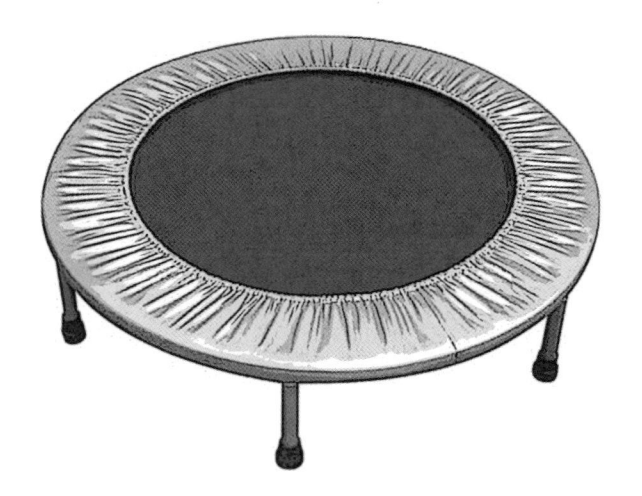

Start/Stop

Individuals with autism tend to have one pace — CONSTANT MOVEMENT or NO MOVEMENT! Start/stop is designed to help the individual with autism know how to change from high gear to stop to cruise to first gear to stop. Changing speed according to the demands of the moment is a beginning step in BODY AWARENESS/BODY CONTROL. One excellent example is toilet training. Toilet training is starting and stopping an activity within the body. School, social situations, jobs and life require starting and stopping appropriately. We have numerous examples of individuals with autism whose toilet training went into high gear once the body learned to start, stop and change speeds. How do you do this?

NOTE: If the individual with autism is always in high gear, start fast. If the individual prefers to sit, start very slow. BEGIN WHERE THEY ARE!

Use one or two helpers for this activity depending on the size of the individual with autism. Taking the arm of the child with autism, move and say:
- Run, run, run, stop! (while you physically move and then stop the child)
- Run, run, run, run, run, stop! (change the length of time you move)
- Run, stop!
- Run, run, walk, walk, stop (change speed)

For the child who is less active, sedentary or physically challenged:
- Walk, stop!
- Walk very slowly, stop!
- Walk, walk, walk, stop!
- Walk, walk, walk faster, stop!

Ride On An Adult's Shoulders

Have the child with autism ride on the shoulders of an adult. The adult will indicate the speed they are going. The child with autism feels the body movement, as well as the quiet body, of the adult.
- Run, run, run, stop.
- Run, walk, stop.
- Walk, stop, walk, run, stop.

Example - An 18 month old child with autism did one thing well - RUN. His Dad said that this run/stop and changing speeds activity was so critical because, once accomplished, Dad did not always need to have his son in a harness. This activity was the beginning of a controlled child! Dad held his son's hand while they practiced run, run, run, stop. When the son became fatigued, Dad carried his son on his shoulders. Later it was practiced side by side.

Start/Stop For Other Activities

What does this individual with autism choose to do? It might be a certain sound (screaming, humming), a movement pattern (twirling, flicking the fingers in front of the eyes), it doesn't matter. Work on starting and stopping that pattern.

- Sounds
- Movement patterns
- Walking
- Walk on toes
- Rolling
- Creeping
- Marching
- Jumping on a trampoline
- Clapping
- Crawling
- Walk on heels

Example - A ten year old with autism had a certain hum his family disliked and repeatedly yelled for him to STOP! The day I asked him to repeat the sound, stop the sound, repeat, stop, repeat, stop, was also the day his language started to change from one sound to a variety of sounds, more appropriate sounds, even though spoken language has not yet occurred.

Start/Stop Advanced

To advance this activity, add start/stop and changing speed to:
- Walking a maze while touching items or not touching mentioned
- Walking around a chair or table
- Creeping under a table and stopping in the middle
- Walking behind the therapist.
- Walking in front of the therapist
- Walking on the right side of the therapist
- Walking on the left side of the therapist
- Walking with a sibling or peer

Walk patterns to do with start and stop.
- Walk in place, forward, sideways, backward and zigzag.
- Walk with toes out, toes turned in or toes straight ahead.
- Walk on tiptoes or heels.
- Walk with knees lifted high.
- Walk slowly as in a processional.
- Walk as if on ice.
- Walk with legs straight and without bending the knees.
- Walk as in a parade.
- Walk while slowly lowering and raising the body.
- Walk while turning, twisting stretching or curling the body.
- Walk fast with long steps or very tiny steps.
- Walk leaning forward or back as if walking up a hill or down a hill.

A person who begins to control his/her body has begun to gain control of his/her world.

Walking Rail

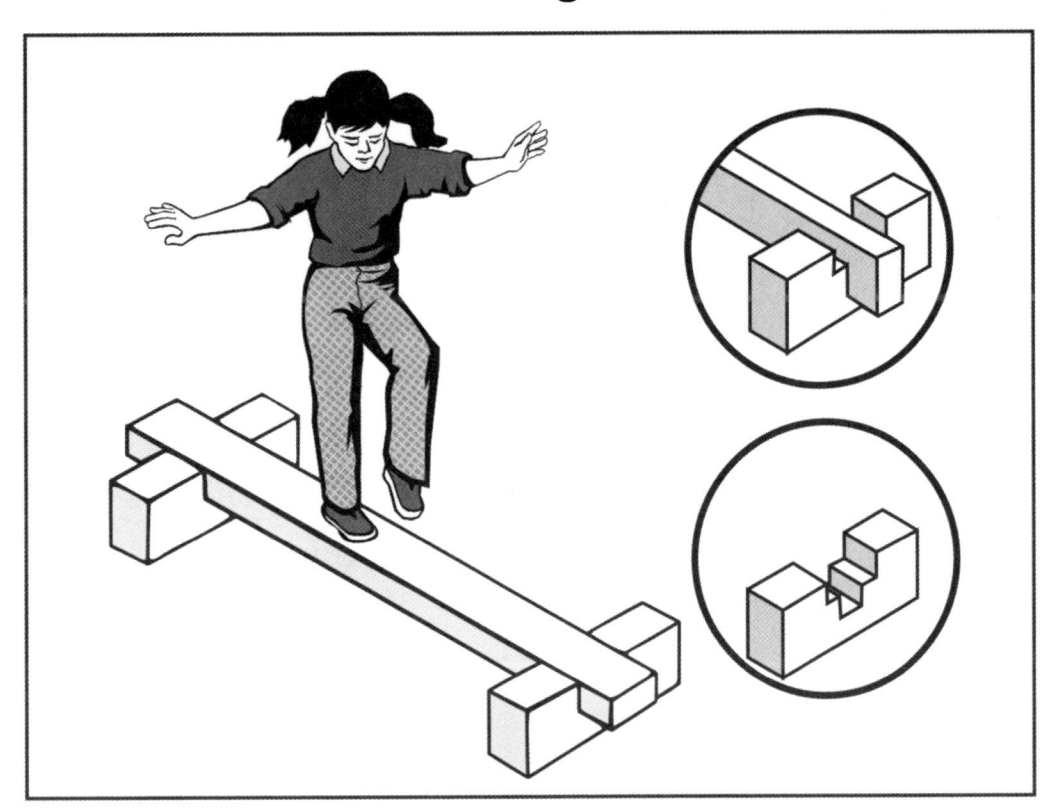

Purpose: How many ways can you walk using the board to enhance balance?

Equipment: 2 X 4 on the floor with support. You can create a walking rail with a 2x4 or purchase a walking rail.

Set-up: Assist child by holding both hands while he/she walks the board forward and backward.

Walking Rail Activities

Begin on the 4" wide of the 2x4 and later go to the 2" side.

1. Holding arms out, walk forward and backward.

2. Holding arms out, walk to the middle, turn around and walk backward.

3. Walk to the middle, turn and walk sideways with weight on the balls of the feet.

4. Walk to the middle, turn and continue sideways right.

5. Walk forward and backward with the left foot in front of the right.

6. Walk forward and backward with the right foot in front of the left.

7. With hands on hips, walk forward and backward.

8. Walk forward and pick up a beanbag from the middle of the board.

9. Walk forward to center, kneel on one knee, stand up and continue.

10. Walk forward and backward with a beanbag balanced on top on head (shoulder, back of hand, or with several beanbags on body parts).

11. Pretend you are an animal (a dog, snake, elephant, giraffe, or rabbit) and move on the rail forward and backward like the animal you are pretending to be.

12. Hop on right foot forward and backward (then left).

13. Walk with arms in different positions (clasped behind the body, clasped on top of head, one arm in front and one in back of the body).

14. Walk holding a weight in both hands, each hand or one hand.

15. The therapist holds a bar 3 inches above the walking rail, walk and step over the bar. Change the height of the bar and repeat. Do with beanbag on head, shoulder, etc., while walking forward, sideways, backward.

16. With bar four feet above the walking rail, walk and duck under the bar. Change height on the bar.

17. Walk forward and backward with eyes opened/closed repeating many of the patterns listed.

18. Walk forward and backward with eyes constantly closed repeating many of the patterns listed.

19. Walk forward and backward while hitting a hanging ball.

20. Walk forward and backward while juggling.

21. Walk forward and backward while singing, counting, doing math, spelling or reviewing for a test.

22. Walk forward and backward while combining spelling and juggling, etc.

Add Rhythm on Walking Rail

1. The therapist sings or chants a song based on what the child is doing. Be sure your singing in beat with the child's movements.

    "Jay is walking on the Walking Rail", "Jay will push the balloon as he walks on the Walking Rail."

2. Sing or chant a song the child likes. Begin by matching the speed of the child. Try changing the speed. If the child moves slowly, change to a slower speed. If the child moves fast, increase the speed of your singing.

3. If a metronome is used, begin at the child's speed before making very small changes.

Add Throwing and Catching
With Bean Bags on Walking Rail

Throw and catch a bean bag or ball while walking.

Walk forward and backward on the Walking Rail while balancing one or more bean bags on a part of the body:

1. Head
2. Back of head
3. Shoulder

Balance Board

Create a balance board that is 12"x30"x1" thick. Pre-drill and drywall screw a 12" length of 2"x 4" board in the center of the board, parallel to the short sides. You may choose to glue a piece of carpeting on top.

1. The therapist moves the board to have each side touch the floor while child maintains balance.

2. Sit in the middle of the board with feet on the floor. Rock the board back and forth with the ends softly touching the floor. Keep the body straight as the board shifts.

3. As you sit with your feet on the floor, balance the board with your hands in various positions.

4. Stand and walk from end to end of the board forward and backward with arms in various positions.

5. Stand on the board with feet as far apart as your shoulders. Shift the board back and forth gently touching the floor. Do in rhythm.

6. Change the foot position; Feet touching in the middle of the board, one foot in the middle and one at the end. Find as many foot variations as possible while maintaining balance.

7. Eye hand coordination and balance: bounce and catch, bounce back and forth, juggle, dribble.

8. Balance and think — involves: balance and do math, spelling, counting, reviewing for a test, or talking.

9. Balance, eye-hand coordination and thinking.

10. Repeat any of the above with eyes closed.

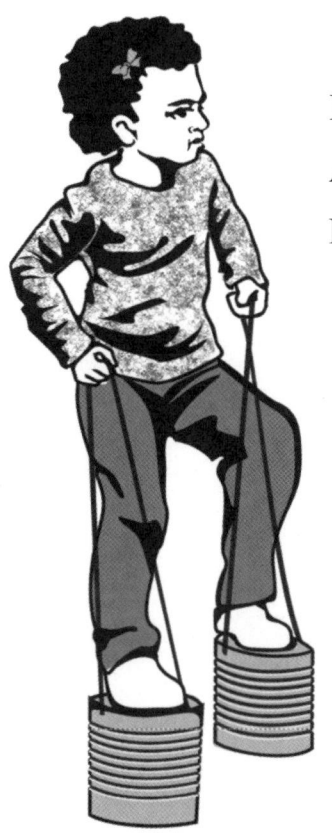

Stilts

Equipment: Number 10 cans or coffee can, ropes.

Attach rope to cans.

Hold onto the ropes and walk standing on the cans.

Judge Distance

Purpose: To learn to judge distance visually. How Far?

Estimate or guess distance while walking to a tree, the corner, a chair.
- How far away is the tree/corner/chair?
- How many steps will it take to get there?
- How many big steps will it take to get there?

Walk to the object (tree, corner, chair etc.) and see if your judgement was correct.

Walk a Road:

Use a string or a rope to create a road.
1. Walk the road forward and back.
    a. Feet on each side of the string.
    b. Heel to toe on the string.
    c. Cross over.
        - Right foot on left side and left foot on the right side.

2. Judge Distance:
    a. Indicate how many steps it would take to get to the corner.
        - Check to see if you were correct.
    b. Vary steps (large or small).

3. Indicate which way to turn:
    - Right or left when reaching the corner.
    - From the corner, turn left.

4. Direct another person around a road maze:
    - When you get to the corner, turn right.

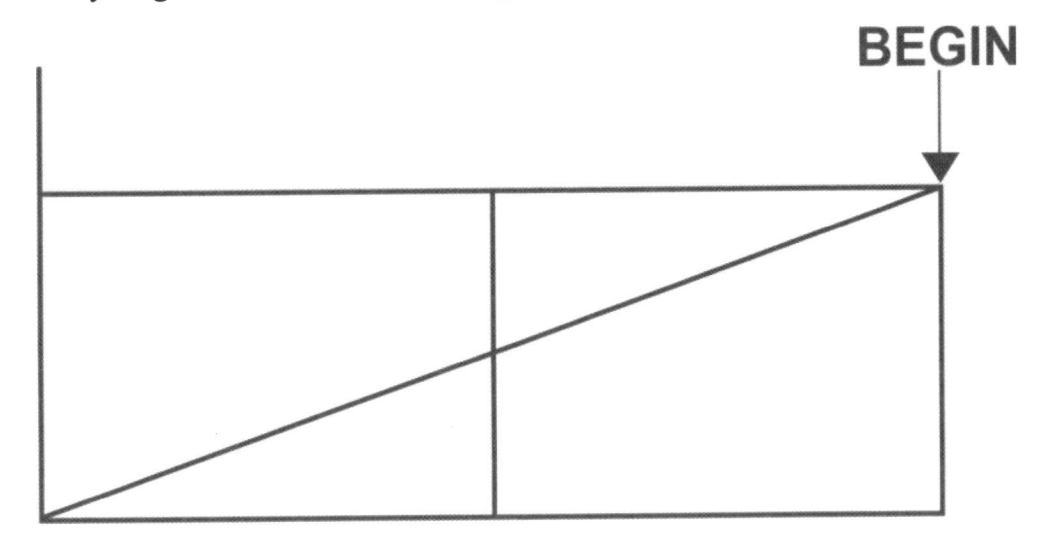

BEGIN

Body Image

Body image comes through awareness.

Body awareness is accomplished through identification of body parts and then movement of parts until this can be done effortlessly.

1. Body Parts - learn the body parts, location, function and relationship to each other.

   Suggested body parts to be learned:

Head	Chin	Waist	Palms
Hair	Mouth	Hips	Fingers
Eyes	Forehead	Legs	Knees
Eyelashes	Neck	Arms	Ankles
Eyebrows	Shoulders	Eyebrows	Heels
Ears	Chest	Wrists	Feet
Nose	Back	Hands	Toes
Cheeks	Abdomen	Soles	

2. Stand facing the child and give the following directions with actions:
   a. Watch me and listen. Touch the parts of your body I tell you to touch with both hands."

   b. Tell me what you are touching.

3. Ask:

   a. What do you see with, bite with, eat with, hear with?

   b. Touch your corresponding body part.

   c. Name that part.

4. Variations:

   a. Have the child perform the tasks while standing in front of a full-length mirror.

   b. Point to the body parts of the person working with you.

   c. Point out the body parts an a doll.

   d. Point out body parts on a picture.

e. Touch body parts to an object - ball, wall, floor.

> Example: Place your foot on a chair, right, left.
> Place your hand on a chair, right, left.

ADD more directions as successful.

f. Keep a balloon in the air by hitting it with the body part named by the therapist.

5. a. Lie down on a large piece of paper. Draw an outline around the body.
Color the figure to represent self.
Dress with cloth or colored paper.

b. Draw a picture of yourself. If a mirror is available, compare the drawing with a mirror image.

c. On a large picture of a person, pin, tape, post-it note or press some type of marker to each body part as it is named.

d. Demonstrate various body positions using a jointed figure such as a doll or wood mannequin (or make segmented figures out of heavy construction paper, using paper fasteners, attaching the segments together at the joints). Instruct the child to arrange a second figure in the same position as directed or as demonstrated.

e. Discuss the bone structure of the body, then draw a skeleton.

f. Make a composite face or body from the features of many pictures.

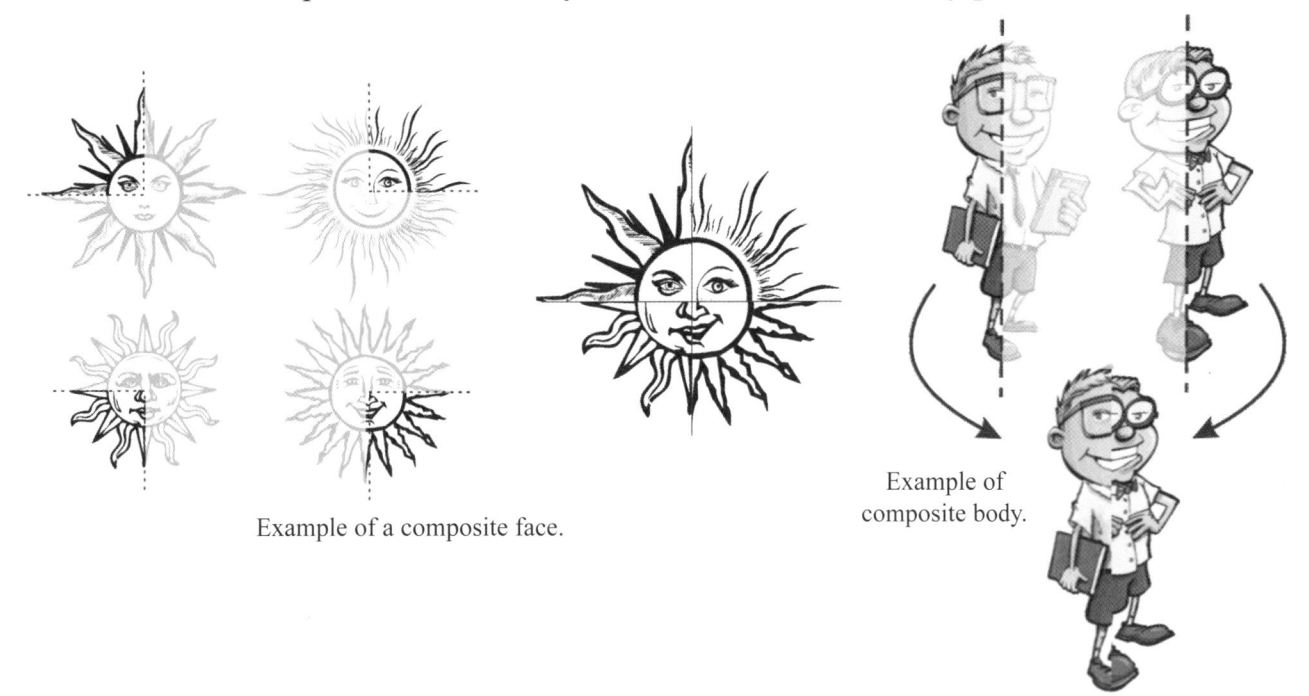

Example of a composite face.

Example of composite body.

Eye-Foot and Eye-Hand Coordination

Purpose: To teach the use of the parts of the body in harmony: eye-foot and eye-hand coordination, visual attention, memory, sequencing and balance.

Equipment:
1. Items to hit
   a. Wiffle balls (3 sizes) hanging by a string (orange or yellow)
   b. Ball on a string (orange or yellow)
2. Dowel - 36" long, 1" - 2" diameter with a variety of colored stripes
3. Balance or twist boards
4. Music

Set-Up:
1. Hang the ball from the ceiling or a light fixture:
   a. 16" above the child lying on his/her back.
   b. Between shoulder and eye level for the child who is sitting.
   c. Between eye and waist height for the child who is standing.
2. Body Positions:
   a. Lie on back looking up at the ball with a straight body.
   b. Sit on a chair or sit pretzel style on the floor within arm's distance of the balloon or ball.
   c. Stand comfortably - feet shoulders-width apart, within arms reach of the ball.

Procedure:

1. Have the child lie on his/her back looking up at the ball:
   a. Hit the ball with one hand - repeat.
   b. Hit the ball with the other hand - repeat.
   c. Hit the ball with alternating hands.
   d. Hit in patterns (two with right, one with left; right, left, right) repeat a pattern many times before going to a new pattern.
   e. Hit gently/soft.
   f. Hit hard.
   g. Hit in patterns, i.e., gently . . . hard . . . gently . . . hard, etc.

2. Sit on chair or pretzel style and repeat.

3. Stand and repeat.

4. Add balance or twist board and repeat.

5. Sit on a chair or the floor and
   a. hit with each hand alone.
   b. hit alternating hands.
   c. hit gentle and hard.
   d. hit in patterns (gentle, hard patterns and right, left patterns).

Dowel

NOTE: Hold the dowel horizontally across the front of the body, one hand on each end of the dowel and shoulder-width distance between the hands. The thumbs are under the dowel. Do the following activities sitting and then repeat the activities while standing.

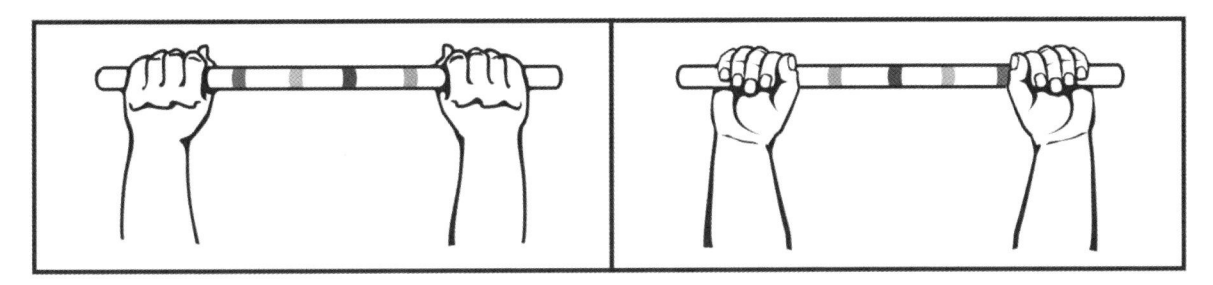

1. Push a hanging ball or balloon gently on one stripe (red or yellow).

2. Add rhythm (follow music from a radio). Push in rhythm to the music.

3. Push on different stripes.

4. Push on the directed stripes (memory patterns).
   a. (red, yellow, red, yellow).
   b. (red, yellow, blue, red, yellow, blue).

5. Hit on the directed stripes with rhythm.

6. Hit while talking, singing, spelling, doing math.
   a. add rhythm.
   b. add memory patterns.

7. The child creates his/her own memory patterns.
   a. add rhythm.
   b. add math problems, spelling, singing.

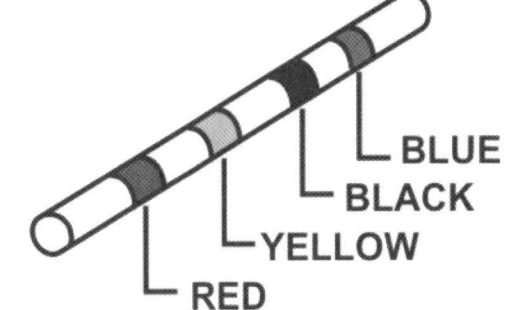

Add Balance

Stand on a balance board or twisting board and repeat the previous patterns.

Eye-Hand - With A Friend

Work sitting or standing or on a balance board, create games with a friend. Play catch:

1. Seated:
    You push the ball to the friend and the friend pushes the ball back to you.
    Standing or on balance board:
    You throw the ball to the friend and the friend throws the ball back to you.

2. Each has a dowel.
    "If I hit the ball on the red stripe, you hit on the red stripe."

3. Create new games with each other.

Roll Balls

Begin with the size ball that the child will work with successfully. Decrease the size of the balls with success. You may begin by moving the hand or foot of the child. Sit on the floor and roll the ball. Aim the ball at one of the therapist's feet, then the other, to one hand, then the other. The therapist returns the ball, aiming at the child's corresponding body part. Instruct the child to push the ball back with:

1. Both hands.
2. Right hand.
3. Left hand.
4. Right foot.
5. . Left foot.

Roll On The Table

Roll the ball across the table and instruct the child to:

1. Stop it with his/her whole hand.

2. Stop it with one finger of each hand.

3. Stop the ball from the top rather than blocking in front of the ball.

4. Roll back and forth, alternating hands.

5. Roll to different places on the table.

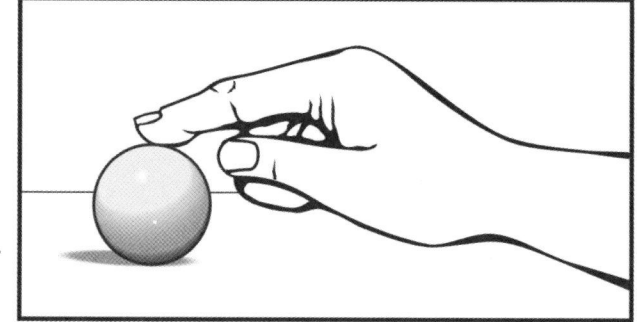

6. Roll the ball, aiming so that it will hit a block, the therapist's hand, or finger that changes position.

7. Roll and knock over blocks in stacks of varying heights and configurations, i.e., towers, walls, etc., placed randomly around the table.

Other Eye-Hand Coordination Tasks

1. **Nuts and bolts**
    Equipment: nuts and bolts of various sizes
    Match the sizes and put the nuts and bolts together.

2. **Pounding**
    Equipment: block of wood, nails, hammer
    a. Pound nails in a random pattern.
    b. Create a shape with the nails.

3. **Drop the clothespin**
    Equipment: clothespins and bottle
    Drop the clothespin in the bottle while:
    a. Kneeling on a chair.
    b. Standing on a chair.
    c. Switching hands.

4. **Piles**
    Equipment: wooden blocks, poker chips, paper cups
    a. Pile as high as possible.
    b. Create a design.

5. **String beads**
    Equipment: beads of different colors and shapes, string
    String beads:
    a. At random.
    b. At random and as fast as possible.
    c. According to a color named.
    d. Design the same pattern another has created.

6. **Lite Brite**
    a. Place the pegs randomly using alternate hands - right, left, right, left.
    b. Place the pegs in a pattern - yellow, red, yellow, red.

7. **Create matching patterns using**
    a. Blocks.
    b. Household items (spoons, toothpicks, coins).
    c. Vary positions in relationship to the child.
       - front, right, left, beside

8. **Sort**
    a. By size - noodles (pasta), nuts and bolts, beans
    b. By colors - blocks, beads

Bean Bags

Purpose: Bean bag activities help develop:

- Balance
- Eye-hand coordination
- Total body coordination
- Directionality (right-left awareness)
- Memory
- Sequencing
- Visualization (getting mental images)
- Peripheral awareness
- Dimensional awareness
- Judging distances
- Eye movement control
- Eye flexibility
- Eye pointing
- Eye shifting

Body Awareness

1. Put the bean bag on your head and walk, sit, hop, run, and jump.

2. Put a bean bag on your head and another on your shoulder and walk, stand on one foot, balance and walk a line.

3. Put three bean bags on your body and move (example: on shoulder, head, and hand).

4. Put bean bags on various parts of your body and see how many things you can do without losing the bean bags.

5. Put a bean bag on your head and see if you can keep it there for an entire day.

Drop The Bean Bag

1. Hold one hand high and one hand low. Drop the bean bag from the high hand to the low hand. If the right hand was high, switch and put the left hand high.

2. Make the distance between the hands greater. Drop the bean bag from one hand to the other. Switch hands. Have the right hand on top and then the left.

3. Stand - put boxes close around your body. Drop the bean bags into the boxes. At times you may have to move the feet.

4. Move the boxes farther away from you. Again, get the bean bags into the boxes. Do not leave your position. Sometimes you can move in a circle and at other times twist the body without moving the feet.

Throw And Catch

Instruct the child to:

1. Throw a bean bag up with both hands AND:
    a. Catch it with both hands
    b. Catch with the right hand
    c. Catch with the left hand

2. Throw a bean bag up with the right hand AND:
    Repeat a. through c above.

3. Throw a bean bag up with the left hand AND:
    Repeat a. through c above.

Instruct the child to:

Throw the bean bag into the air so that when the bean bag comes down, it will hit:

    the child's hand (both, right, left)

    the child's foot (both, right, left)

    the child's head

    the child's back

    the child's stomach

    the child's shoulders (right and left)

    the child's wrist (right and left)

    the child's knee (right and left)

    the child's hip (right and left)

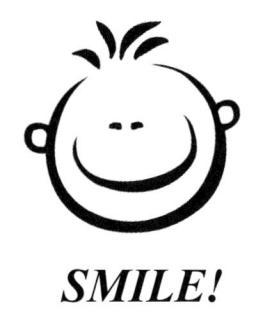

Throw A Bean Bag At A Stationary Target

Put boxes or pails at different distances from your body.

1. Throw overhand and get the bean bag into the box or pail.
    a. Throw with both hands
    b. Throw with the right hand
    c. Throw with the left hand

2. Throw underhand and get the bean bag into the box or pail.
    Repeat a. through c. above.

3. Throw sidearm and get the bean bag into the box or pail.
    Repeat a. through c. above.

How Far Away???

Throw the bean bag and get it a certain distance from the pail or box. Take a ruler or a piece of string to mark the distance. What distance will you choose? Example: I will get the bean bag one foot away and on the right side of the box.

1. Throw overhand and get a certain predetermined distance from the target (i.e. one inch).
    a. Throw with both hands
    b. Throw with the right hand
    c. Throw with the left hand

2. Throw underhand and get a certain predetermined distance from the target (i.e. one foot).
    Repeat a. through c above.

3. Throw sidearm and get a certain predetermined distance from the target (i.e. three inches).
    Repeat a. through c above.

4. Throw a bean bag to the ceiling and have the bean bag touch the ceiling GENTLY.
    Repeat a. through c above.

5. Throw the bean bag CLOSE to the ceiling WITHOUT hitting the ceiling.
    Repeat a. through c above.

Throw And Move

1. Throw the bean bag into the air, sit down on the floor or on a chair and catch the bean bag.

2. Throw the bean bag into the air from a sitting position, stand and catch the bean bag.

3. Throw the bean bag up into the air, turn and catch the bean bag.

4. Throw the bean bag from behind your back to in front of you and catch it.

5. Throw the bean bag under the leg and catch (right and left).

WOW!!

Throw And Clap Or Slap

1. Throw the bean bag into the air, clap one time and catch the bean bag.
    a. Clap two times
    b. Clap three times

2. Throw the bean bag into the air, clap one time and slap your knees before catching.
    a. Clap two times and slap one time
    b. Clap one time and slap two times
    c. Invent your own patterns

Remember to throw with both hands, right hand and left hand at different times.

Dot To Dot, Bean Bag To Bean Bag

Place one bean bag on the floor.

Place two bean bags in another location.

Place three or four bean bags in still another location.

Instruct the child to walk to the group of three bean bags and then to the group of four bean bags and finally to the group with one bean bag. Create different patterns.

Breathing

Lie on your back. Put one bean bag on your waist and another on your chest. Your diaphragm is located at your waist. As you breathe, your diaphragm is to move and NOT your chest.

Take a deep breath. The bean bag at your waist should move up or your stomach should appear to get bigger as the air enters your body. The bean bag on your chest should not move.

EXHALE or slowly let the air leave your body. The bean bag at your waist should go down as the air leaves your body. Keep practicing. The bean bag on your chest is to remain still. The bean bag at your waist goes up as you take a breath and down as the air leaves your body.

Deep Breathing Helps You Stay Relaxed!!

Bean Bag On Your Head Trick

When reading, writing, walking or watching TV keep that bean bag on your head to be sure you are sitting very tall and keeping your head horizontally level. Try this for a full day or several days to become very aware of your posture. Correct posture is important for your eyes, spine, breathing and your general health.

Balloon Activities

Purpose: To teach eye-foot and eye-hand coordination.

Consider: The eyes learn to pay attention by following a moving target. A balloon is a good target to begin with since it is slow in speed and does not hurt if it hits you.

Equipment: Round balloon - bright in color
Balance board or twist board
Trampoline
Walking Rail
Ping Pong Paddles
Badminton racquets

Hanging Balloon

Fill the balloon with water to about half full, then blow up the balloon and tie the end. Attach to a string and hang it from the ceiling or light fixture so that the position of the balloon is just touching the floor for eye-foot coordination or between eye and waist level for eye-hand coordination.

CAUTION: Balloons are NOT to be in the mouth. Be especially concerned with pieces of balloons. A partially blown balloon will not break as easily as a tightly blown balloon.

Eye-Foot Coordination

Many individuals with autism find eye-hand coordination stressful. Begin with eye-foot coordination activities. Body position for eye-foot activities is sitting on a chair with feet flat on the floor. You may need to show the child sitting in the chair how to move their legs. Have the child wear a shoe on one foot and a sock on the other to feel the different sides. If this doesn't work, try a different color sock on each foot or tape different pictures or stickers on the top of the child's shoes.

1. Push the balloon
   a. with the right foot alone.
   b. with the left foot alone.
   c. alternating right and left feet.

2. Push the balloon
   a. hard then soft with the right foot alone
   b. hard then soft with the left foot alone
   c. hard then soft, alternating right and left feet.
      in hard/soft patterns (i.e.: "2 hard, 3 soft" or "hard - soft - hard - soft," etc.).
   d. aiming so the balloon touches the therapist standing opposite the child

36

Eye-Hand Coordination

Body positions for eye-hand activities are:
- Sitting on the floor or in a chair.
- Lying on back, looking up at the balloon.
- Standing.
- Balancing on a balance board.

1. Push the balloon with
   a. the right hand alone.
   b. the left hand alone.
   c. alternate hands.

2. Push the balloon hard/soft with
   a. the right hand.
   b. the left hand.
   c. alternate hands.
   d. hard/soft pattern, i.e., 2 hard . . . 1 soft . . . 2 hard . . . 1 soft, etc.

3. Push the balloon in patterns
   a. right hand, left hand, right hand, left hand.
   b. right, right, left; right, right, left.
   c. right, left, left; right, left, left.

4. Push the balloon to touch the therapist's
   a. hand.
   b. stomach.
   c. back.

5. Add the ping pong paddles.
   a. Push the balloon using a ping pong paddle held in the dominant hand, keeping the non-dominant hand down close to the side of the body.
   b. Switch the ping pong paddle to the non-dominant hand, keeping the dominant hand down close to the side of the body.
   c. Holding ping pong paddles in each hand, push the balloon, alternating left – right – left –right, etc.

Add Rhythm

Turn on a radio, CD player or metronome. Often individuals with autism have favorite music they listen to. If not already with them, ask the parents to bring the child's favorite music to use in establishing rhythm for the activity being done.

1. Push the balloon in rhythm on the beat of the music (or metronome).

2. Push the balloon off the beat.

3. Push the balloon in rhythm and in patterns.

> Example: Push the balloon in rhythm with the beat, "push - skip a beat - push - skip a beat," or "push - push - skip a beat - push - push -skip a beat," etc.

Add Balance with the Balance Board

Have the child stand on the balance board. The upper body should remain motionless, bending at the knees and hips, alternating left leg then right leg to shift balance from side to side. The therapist may need to physically move the knees to show the child how to do this activity. (This may require two people to help in the beginning - one to hold the child steady and the second to physically bend the knees. Later, have the child put his/her hands on the therapist's shoulders while the therapist physically moves the knees).

1. Shift balance so that the opposite sides of the board touch the floor.
2. Balance weight evenly on the board so that neither side touches the floor.
3. Balance while moving one arm in different positions - up, down, out, in, in circles, sides of the body, in front of the body. Then repeat the same movements with the other arm, and then both arms in unison.
4. While balancing, push the hanging balloon, alternating hands.
5. While balancing, push the free floating balloon, alternating hands.
6. While balancing, bounce/catch a ball using both hands, then each hand alone, then alternating hands.
7. While balancing, dribble a ball. Begin with a larger ball (approximately 9"). Continue, making the ball smaller with the child's success.
8. As the child progresses, add singing, counting and spelling to the above activities for multitasking.

Add Balance with the Walking Rail

Walk a walking rail forward and back while you:

   a. push the balloon.

   b. push the balloon in patterns, i.e., to the right; to the left.

   c. push the balloon in patterns while singing.

   d. push the balloon to the beat of a metronome, beginning at the child's speed.

   e. Increase the speed of the metronome slowly.

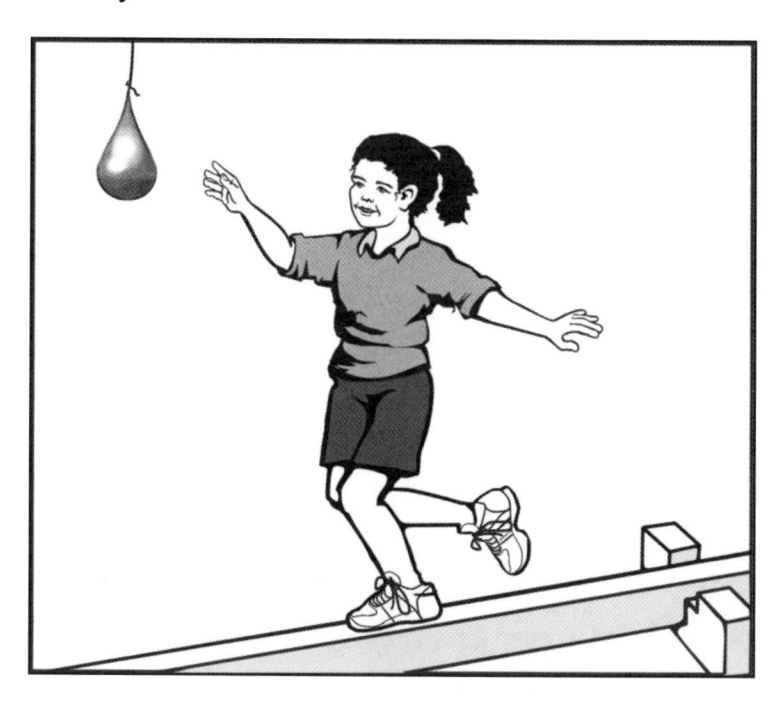

Moving Target & Moving Individual - Trampoline

1. Jump on the trampoline and
    a. push the balloon with each hand.
    b. push the balloon in patterns (left, left, right).
    c. push the balloon in patterns to rhythm while chanting what the child is doing at the child's rhythmic speed.
    d. push the balloon in patterns off the beat.

2. Jump your feet in patterns on the trampoline (apart - together; apart - together)
    a. Make the foot patterns harder.
       - One foot in front, switch.
       - Two hops right, one left.
       - 1...2...2...1
    b. Jump your feet in patterns and play balloon volleyball.

Free Floating Balloon

Go back to the first balloon activity. This time you are working with a free floating balloon that is not filled with water. The goal is to keep the feet stationary. (The trampoline activities require jumping, of course.)

1. Push the balloon upwards to the ceiling.
2. Push the balloon in continually more complicated patterns. (i.e., 2 right, 1 left)
3. Push the balloon upwards hard and soft in patterns. (i.e., 2 hard right, 1 soft left)
4. Push the balloon upwards in rhythm while counting number of hits.
5. Add balance.
6. Add the trampoline.

Add Math

Have the child count with each push of the balloon.
1. Count 1 to 10 and back to 1.
2. Count by 10's to 100 and back to 10.
3. Count by 5's to 50 and back to 5.
4. Count by 2's to 20 and back to 2.
5. Count by 3's to 30 and back to 3.
6. Count by 4's, 6's, 7's, 8's and back.

Add Singing

Most individuals with autism enjoy music. Use the rhythm of a favorite song or create a song using the child's name - "Dylan is hitting the balloon, hitting the balloon, hitting the balloon." The child's speed and accuracy determines the speed of the song or chant.

Balloon Volleyball or Tennis

This has become one of the favorite activities for those with or without autism, Before you begin, create a "net" in the center of the room using string, a walking rail, chair or any obstacle that will divide the space into two sections.

1. Instruct the child to push the balloon, using alternating hands, to the person across the "net": Keep the balloon going back and forth as long as possible.

2. Add ping pong paddles.
    a. Begin with one paddle in the dominant hand with the non-dominant hand empty. Push the balloon across the "net", alternating hands, i.e., with the paddle hand - without the paddle hand.
    b. Switch the paddle to the non-dominant hand, leaving the dominant hand empty. Push the balloon to the person across the "net," alternating hands as before.
    c. Now use paddles in both hands, pushing the balloon across the net in an alternating pattern.

3. Add badminton racquets. Note: As the child switches from empty hands to ping pong paddles to badminton racquets, the child is learning depth perception or, "where is the item in relationship to my body?"
    a. Begin with a badminton racquet in the dominant hand and a ping pong paddle in the non-dominant hand. Push the balloon to the person across the "net," alternating hands left, then right, etc.
    b. Switch the badminton racquet to the non-dominant hand and the ping pong paddle to the dominant hand, and continue pushing the balloon over the net in an alternating pattern, left - right, etc.
    c. Now use badminton racquets in each hand. Repeat pushing the balloon with alternating hands.
    d. Push the balloon over the net using only one badminton racquet in the dominant hand and leaving the non-dominant hand empty.
    e. Switch the badminton racquet to the non-dominant hand, leaving the dominant hand empty.

Balloon Volleyball On The Trampoline

The child jumps on the trampoline and pushes the balloon to therapist/parent. The child pushes the balloon back and forth as many times as possible.

Example 1: Push the hanging balloon as many times as possible in a row.

Example 2: Jump on the trampoline with a foot pattern of feet apart/feet together while hitting the floating balloon in a pattern all done to rhythm while counting by 6's.

Other Balloon Games

1. Push a balloon into the air with a wooden paddle, a paper plate or a cardboard cylinder.

2. Rebound the balloon off a wall.

3. Push the balloon with different parts of the body.

4. Balloon volley - volley the balloon back and forth between one another. Try to keep the balloon in the air, first with the right hand, then left hand, right foot, etc., using elbow, knees, top of head - anything you can think of.

Soap Bubbles

Equipment: Soap bubbles, wand

1. Blow bubbles, catch and break between hands.

2. Step on the bubble as it hits the floor.

3. Catch on the right hand then the left hand.

4. Catch on the wand.

5. Poke the bubble with a finger on your right hand next your left hand.

Dribbling

Purpose: Develop eye-hand coordination.
Improve near-far shifting of the eyes.
Enhance eye movement control.

Equipment: Balls of various sizes, balance - twist boards, recording paper or calendar

Procedure:

1. Begin with the smallest ball you can successfully dribble.
    a. Dribble with your dominant hand - record the number of dribbles.
    b. Dribble with your non-dominant hand - record the number of dribbles.
    c. Dribble with alternate hands - record the number of dribbles.

2. Work to improve the number of dribbles you can do at one time until you get to 100. THEN...

3. Switch to a smaller ball. When the size of the ball is 2" or smaller, use fewer fingers UNTIL...

4. You can dribble a tiny ball with one finger 100 times.

5. Continue working with this activity to keep the eyes and hands working in a flexible manner.

Increase Difficulty By Moving And Dribbling

Note: Individuals with autism may need to begin with.

1. Bounce and catch the ball.
2. Bounce, hit, catch.
3. Increase number of hits until dribbling is achieved.

Once dribbling has been achieved:

1. Walk and dribble, moving forward and backward.
2. Skip and dribble, moving forward and backward.
3. Dribble while hopping
    - on the dominant foot.
    - on the non-dominant foot.
    - forward and backward.

Dribble to Music

1. Dribble to the beat of the music.
2. Change the music so that you dribble faster or slower.
3. Dribble and move using music.
4. Dribble off the beat of the music.

Add Balance

1. Stand on the balance board while you:
    a. Dribble with the right hand, left hand and alternating hands
    b. Add rhythm.

2. Create a line on the floor using a piece of string..
    a. Dribble over the string.
        - in patterns
        - two on the right and three on the left
        - with rhythm
    b. Change your dribbling.

Add Thinking

1. Dribble and count from 1 to 10 and back 10 to 1.
2. Count by
    a. 10's to 100 and back to 10.
    b. 2's to 20 and back to 2.
    c. 5's to 50 and back to 5.
    d. 3's to 30 and back to 3.
3. Spell words forward and backward.
4. Just talk and dribble.
5. Balance, think and dribble.

Pre-Writing Activities

Remember: **Work for short periods of time, then gradually longer periods of time. This helps prevent frustration.**

Body strength does NOT indicate readiness for writing. Attention, flexibility and control are key elements.

Sticking Hands

1. Using the whole hand
   a. Two individuals maintain hand to hand contact as if the hands were sticking together.
   b. The therapist moves his/her hand while the child maintains contact with his/her hand.
   c. Move in extremes:
      - up, down
      - right, left
      - angles
      - circles
   d. The therapist describes the moves as they occur. "We are moving up."
      - Begin with the dominant hand.
      - Non-dominant hand.
      - Both hands.

2. Finger -repeat sticking using only the index finger.

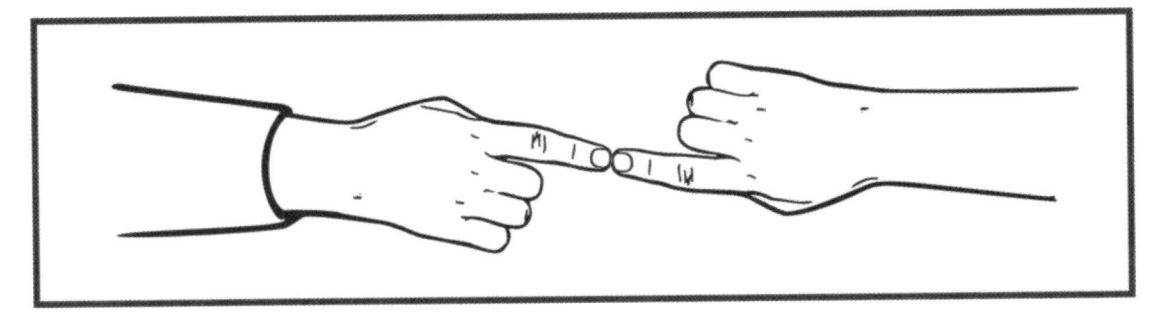

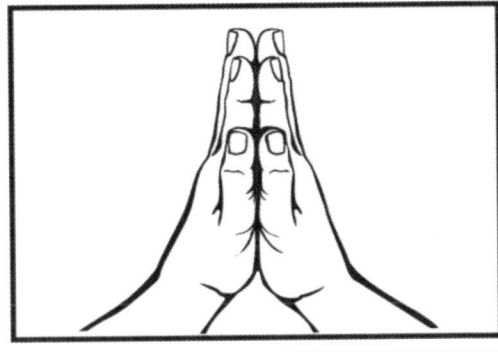

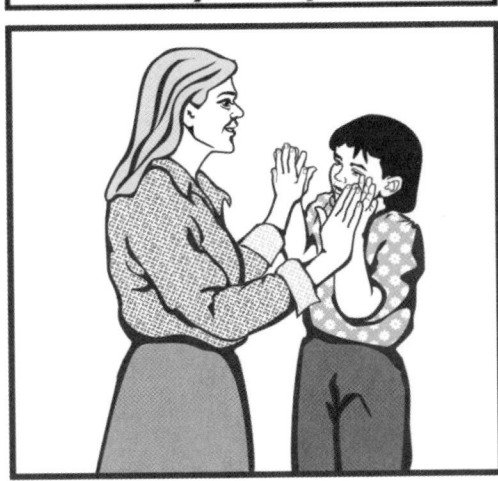

On-off Sticking:

The therapist will "jump" his/her finger/hand to a new location. Note: This is similar to working on a keyboard.

  MOVE:
- a. up, down
- b. right, left
- c. angles
- d. circles or other shapes

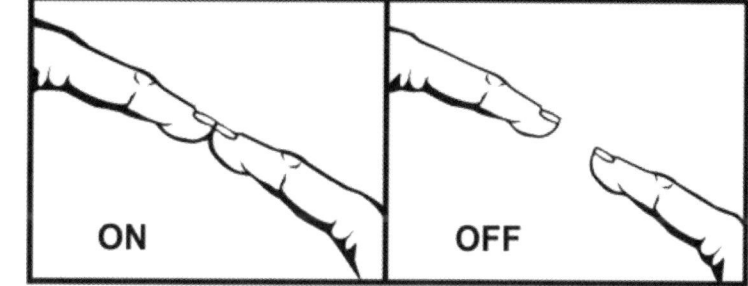

The therapist describes the moves as they occur.
- a. Begin with the dominant hand.
- b. Non-dominant hand
- c. Both hands

Sticking - Pen To Pen

Both the therapist and child have a heavy marking pen with a broad tip. The tips of the pens touch just as you had the fingers touch.

  MOVE:
- a. up, down
- b. right, left
- c. angles
- d. circles or other shapes

  GRIP:
- a. Whole hand grip at first
- b. Three finger grip
- c. Dominant hand
- d. Non-dominant hand

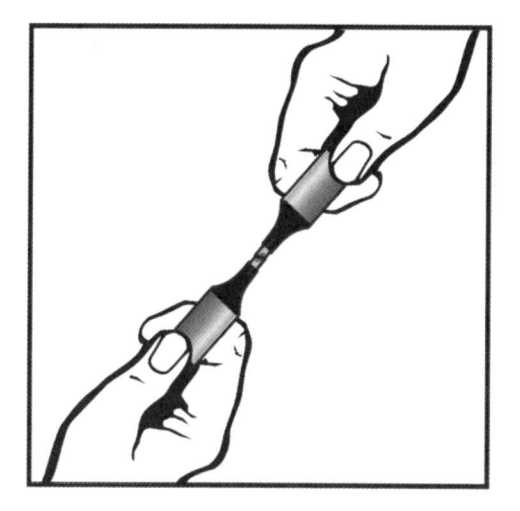

On-off Sticking With Pens

The therapist will "jump" his/her pen to a new location. The child will locate and touch the therapist's pen. Repeat.
- a. Use whole hand grasp
- b. Three finger grasp
- c. Use dominant hand
- d. Use non-dominant hand

Scribble

Encourage scribbling with both hands. Use a chalkboard or large pieces of paper.
- a. Whole hand grasp
- b. Three finger grasp
  - relaxed wrist
  - correct posture
- c. Basic movement patterns
  - up - down
  - right - left
  - angle lines
  - circles
  - start -stop
- d. Fill the entire area with scribbling
  - on a chalkboard
  - on a piece of paper

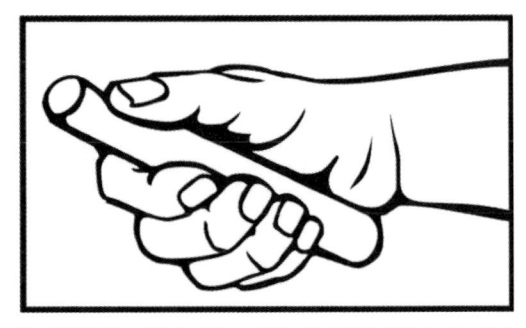

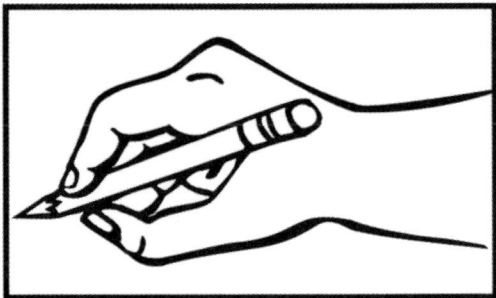

Visual Motor Activity Station

Sticking

The therapist and child sit across from each other at a table or desk. Introduce the Visual Motor Activity Station (VMAS)*, or use a piece of rigid, clear acrylic, plastic or plexiglass held in a vertical position between the therapist and the child.

- a. Using dry erase markers, the therapist draws a shape on one side of the acrylic while the child follows the therapist's pen, drawing on the reverse side at the same time.
- b. The two pens are moving at the same time or sticking.
- c. The therapist describes his/her movement patterns. "We are moving in a circle."
- d. Erase and repeat the task drawing different shapes.

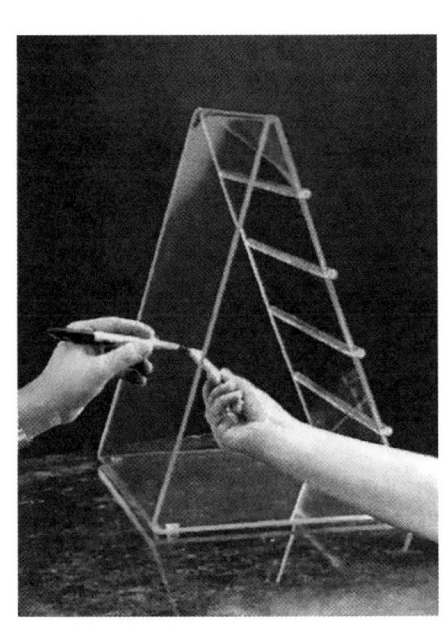

* Visual Motor Activity Station shown in photo was designed by Donna Wendelburg and made by American Acrylics, 108 11th Ave., South Milwaukee, WI 53172. Contact by email at wittmanmike@gmail.com

Off-On Sticking

The therapist will now introduce off-on sticking with the Visual Motor Activity Station. The child's pen touches the therapist's pen with the acrylic in between.

1. Draw shapes, numbers and letters, naming each one as you go.

2. Create pictures, i.e., a house, flower, car, cat, dog, etc.

3. Play follow the leader and discuss where you might go. For example, the therapist says, "Let's go to the library to read a book about dogs." "Now where do you want to go?" The child says, "I want to get a chocolate ice cream cone." Continue the trip.

Jumping

The therapist puts the tip of the marker on the acrylic. The child touches his/her marker to the same spot. The therapist jumps to a new spot and the child follows. Repeat, changing speed. If the child is able to maintain attention, fill the entire area of the acrylic surface.

Tracing

The therapist draws a line with a dry erase marker and the child traces the line and says, "I am making a horizontal line." The therapist draws two lines and the child traces the two lines. Continue with harder shapes.

Draw On Back

1. Using the index finger, the therapist draws a shape (i.e., a circle) on the back of the child and says, "I am making a circle." Instruct the child to draw that shape on the plexiglass (shown placed on a slanted surface) using a dry erase marker.

2. The therapist draws a different shape on the back of the child and on the plexiglass, again stating verbally what shape is being drawn. Instruct the child to trace the shape using his/her finger.

3. Repeat steps using more complex shapes, numbers and letters but without verbal instruction.

Hints for Desk or Table Activities

- Correct posture and furniture sizes are critical in reducing visual and body stress when doing close work. Arms on a chair may be necessary so the child can maintain balance.

- Work on a slanted surface for comfort. The recommended angle of slant is 20°.

- Have excellent lighting with no glare and no shadows. Try incandescent and fluorescent lights to see if the child reacts differently.

- Have PLANNED visual breaks to reduce stress. For example, if the child can work effectively for five minutes, take a break each four minutes and then come back to work. Make the break a movement break (i.e. hitting a balloon or jumping on a trampoline). Increase sitting time and decrease the movement time with success. Know that sitting time may begin with 10 to 15 seconds.

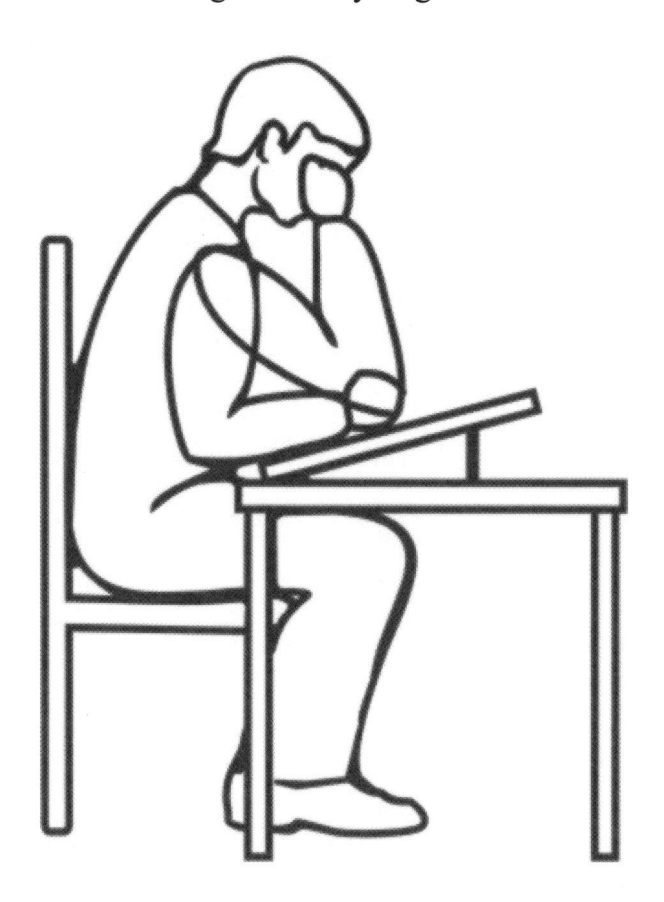

Chalkboard Activities

REMEMBER:
- Use smooth, free-flowing movements.
- Stand back and observe what you have made.
- Follow part of your design with your fingers.

Scribbling

1. Use full arm movements, moving elbow and shoulder rather than just the fingers and wrist.

2. Use each hand independently as well as both hands in unison.

3. Cover the board with chalk and erase with large circular movements using the palms of your hands.

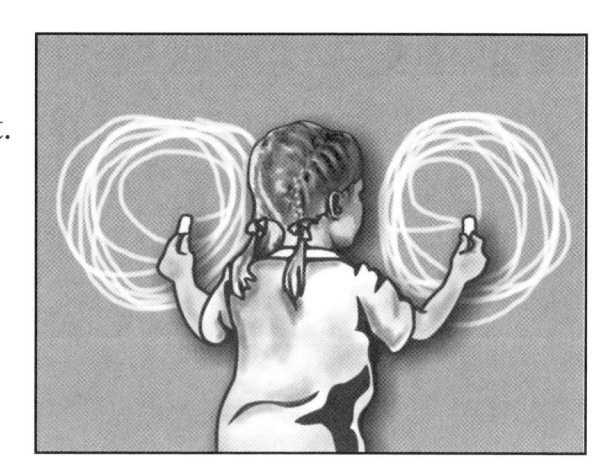

Straight Line Drawing:

The therapist draws two X's on the chalkboard a distance apart. Have the child:

1. Draw a straight line from left X to the right X.

2. Draw a straight line from the right X to the left X.

3. Change hands and repeat the activity.

X _____ X

△ _____ △

Variation: Change the target (example: instead of X's, use triangles as shown).

Two Hands Drawing Two Horizontal Lines

1. Place an X on the board at eye level.

2. Face the X.

3. Using each hand, one on each side of the X, draw horizontal lines away from the midline.

4. Then back again.

5. Repeat the activity and move a given number of times.

L.H. _____ x _____ R.H.

(Left Hand)   (Right Hand)

Multiple Horizontal Lines

L.H.   **R.H.**

_____ X _____
_____ X _____
_____ X _____

1. Eyes on the X (placed at eye level), extend your arms upward and place chalk on the board.
2. Using your hands simultaneously, draw horizontal lines, one under the other.
3. The movement is from the mid-line out.
4. Then the movement may be changed, and the lines are drawn toward the mid-line.
5. Draw using both hands moving from left to right.
6. Draw using both hands moving from right to left.

Multiple Vertical Lines:

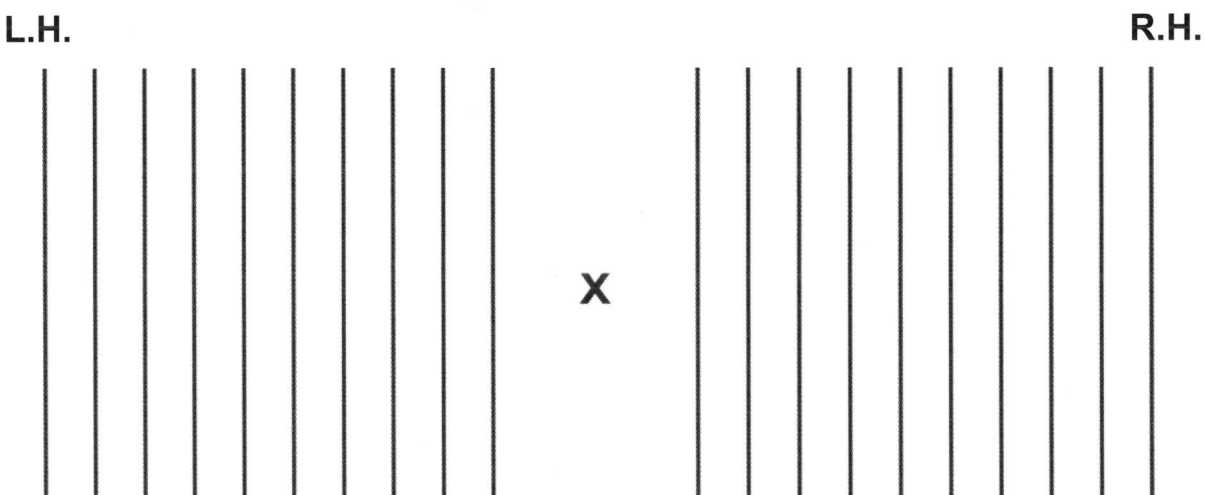

L.H.   **R.H.**

| | | | | | | | | | | X | | | | | | | | | | |

1. Eyes on the X (placed at eye level), starting at your mid-line, draw vertical lines with both hands, as far as each hand will reach to the side
2. Begin at the far point and draw vertical lines, moving toward the mid-line.
3. Starting either at the mid-line or at the outside, draw the lines in an upward movement.

Continuous Vertical Lines

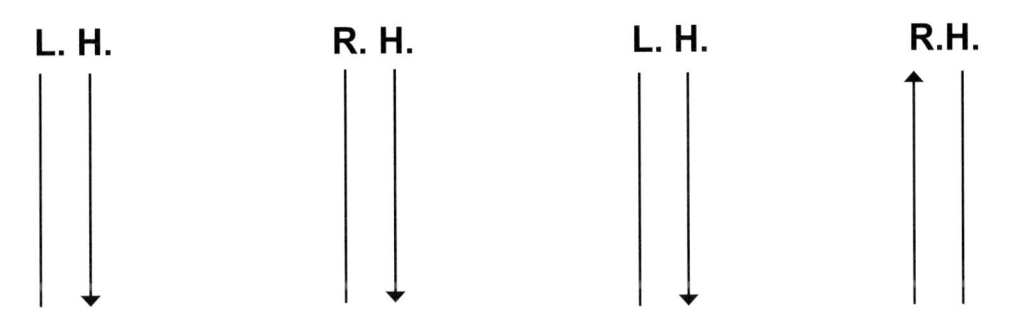

L. H.   **R. H.**   **L. H.**   **R.H.**

1. Reach up and place chalk on the chalkboard.
2. Moving both hands downward, draw a vertical line with each hand.
3. Move hands upward.
4. Continue to move hands in this manner for a designated number of times.
5. Move hands in opposition for a designated number of times.
6. Emphasize easy, rhythmic movement.

One Vertical Line: One Horizontal Line

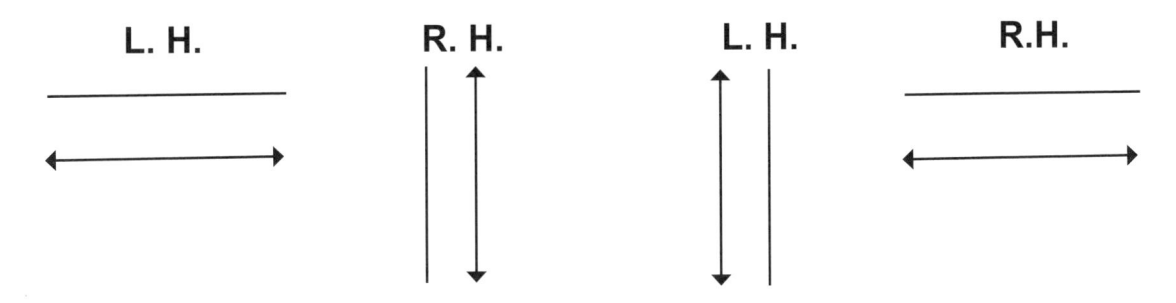

L. H.   **R. H.**   **L. H.**   **R.H.**

1. Moving both hands at the same time, draw one vertical line and one horizontal line.
2. Move the hands continually and rhythmically on these lines for a certain number of times.
3. Repeat the activity but reverse the direction of lines drawn by each hand.

A Circle

1. Draw a circle in front of your face on the chalkboard.
2. Draw a circle by moving your hand in the opposite direction.
3. Change hands and repeat the activity.

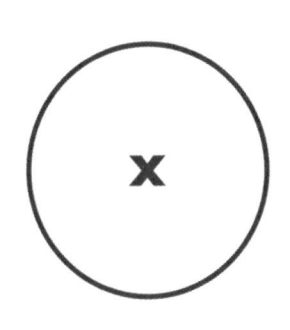

Two Circles

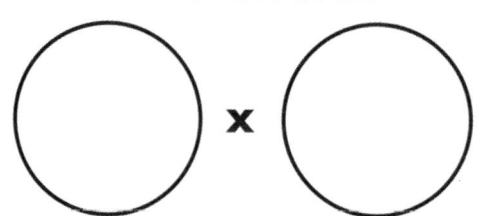

The child stands at the chalkboard with eyes on the X (at eye level), draw two circles simultaneously, hands moving in the direction indicated by the arrows:

1. Left clockwise, right counterclockwise
2. Left counterclockwise, right counterclockwise
3. Left clockwise, right clockwise
4. Left counterclockwise, right clockwise

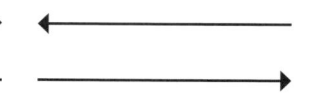

A Square

1. Draw a square in front of your face on the chalkboard
2. Rhythmic movement by counting 1-2-3-4 as the lines are drawn
3. Draw the square moving your hand in the opposite direction
4. Change hands and repeat the activity

Two Squares

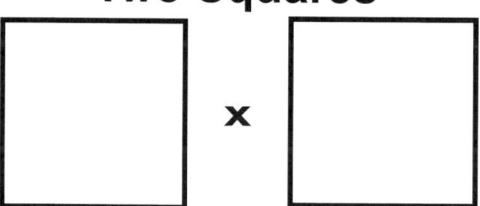

Eyes on the X (at eye level), draw two circles simultaneously, hands moving in the direction indicated by the arrows:

1. Left clockwise, right counterclockwise
2. Left counterclockwise, right clockwise
3. Left clockwise, right clockwise
4. Left counterclockwise, right counterclockwise

A Triangle

1. Eyes on the X (placed at eye level), draw a triangle in front of your face on the chalkboard.
2. Rhythmic movement by counting 1-2-3 as the sides are drawn.
3. Move your hand in the opposite direction.
4. Change hands and repeat the activity.

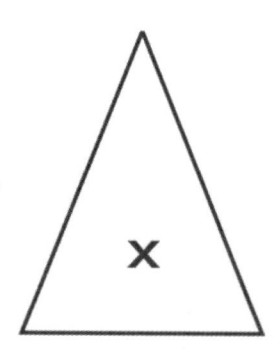

Dots

1. This activity may be done alone or with a partner.
2. The dots are placed at random on the board.
3. The procedure may be: chalk on the dot, eyes on the next dot, bring the chalk to the dot your eyes are viewing.
    a. Draw a line to each dot as soon as it is placed.
    b. All of the dots are placed and then draw a line from one dot to another.
4. Eyes move first to the next dot
    Note: Size of the dots should start large and progressively get smaller.

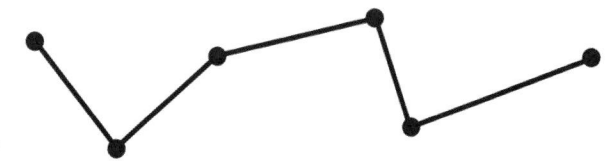

Connecting Forms

1. In this variation of dots, shapes are substituted for the dots.
2. The shapes may be alike or different

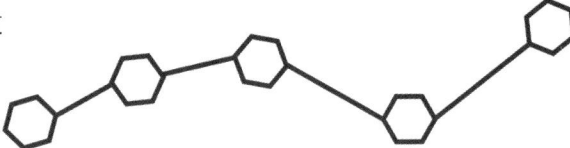

Roadrunner

1. Using a piece of chalk as a car, place your car on the road at the beginning and drive to the end of the road.
2. The eyes lead the hand and chalk.
3. Change direction at the end of the road or on a signal from the therapist. 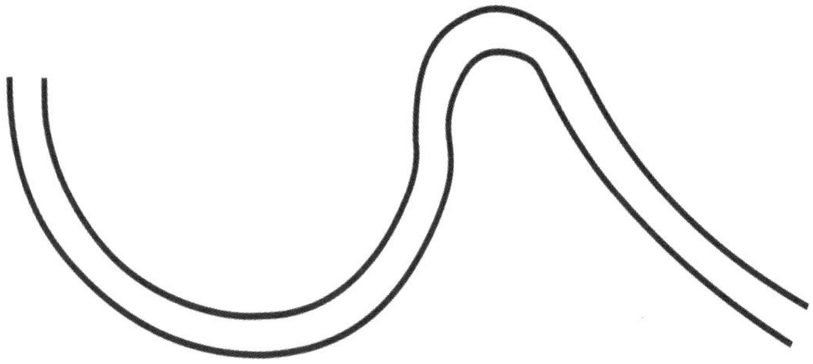
4. If you cannot keep your car on the road, the therapist may have to help you.
5. When your skill improves, do not allow your car to touch the sides of the road.

Racetrack

1. Draw a racetrack on the chalk board.
2. Stand facing the middle of the racetrack.
3. Using a piece of chalk as a car drive the car around the track moving as the arrows indicate.
4. The eyes lead the hand and chalk.
5. Change direction on command. 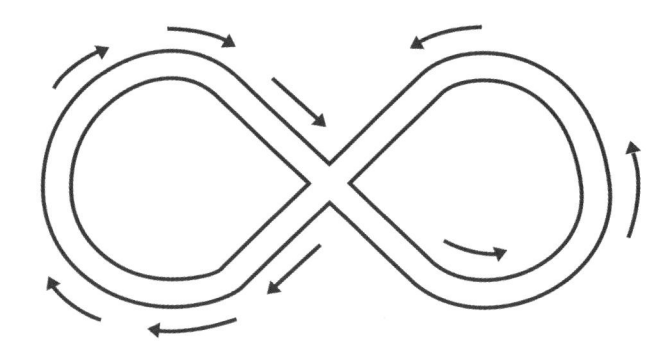
6. Set a certain number of times the car is to be driven around the track.
7. Change hands and repeat the activity.

Teaching Responsibility

Purpose: Develop independence

Develop self esteem

A key element of "maturity" is the ability to accept more responsibility.

Consider: A handicap may change the type of responsibility an individual can handle. A handicap does NOT reduce the importance of being responsible for oneself and learning to help others.

Procedure: Work as a team to complete a task. Continue working as a team until the child can do a part of the task. Give the child more and more of the job until he/she can do the entire task.

Divide Your Tasks:

For the parent to do at home with the child.

Personal
- Take clothes off
- Put clothes on
- Put away "your" things
- Get out clothes to wear
- Brush teeth, comb hair
- Bathe
- Make bed
- Pour milk

With the family
- Put napkins on the table
- Get an apple to eat
- Clean up spills
- Deliver a message

Reaching out to extend the family
- Send a note to a family member.
- Help other people

Reaching out to the world
- Adopt nursing home grandparents
- Give a gift to a stranger (with parental supervision)

Making choices:

Ask what they would like:
- Apple or orange?
- White socks or blue socks?
- Blue jeans or black slacks?
- 1/2 glass of milk or full glass of milk?

Later:
- Which clothes will you wear?
- Which TV show would you like to watch?

Change the expected activities. Too much repetition creates boredom. Boredom is a problem. Have the child help determine activities. Reward for accomplishing tasks.

Remember: **When eye-hand coordination, balance and total body coordination do not match intelligence, acting out behaviors or withdrawal are often the response.**

Print Size

The smaller the print size, the greater the demand on focus. More stress may be encountered by trying to maintain clear vision at desk or at book distances.[9]

	Print Size	Recommended Grade
See the ball.	18 point type	GRADE 1: 14 to 18 point
See the ball.	16 pont type	GRADE 2-3: 14 to 16 point
See the ball.	14 point type	GRADE 2-3: 14 to 16 point
See the ball.	12 point type	GRADE 4: 12 point
See the ball.	10 point type	GRADE 5-8: 10 to 12 point

**Size of print SHOULD NOT be determined by age.
Reduce print size ONLY if the child handles it well.**

TRY

- Large print
- Excellent quality paper
    - plain
    - yellow or canary color
- Bookmark on the TOP of the line being read.

- Encourage eye movement and NOT head movement when reading.

**Some individuals with autism read the entire page with one look.
DO NOT change a successful pattern!**

Observe Behavior for Signs of Stress

A relaxed body allows for a longer attention span. The body exhibits many signs of stress.

Learn To Read The Signs:

Behavior to watch for:

- Head rocking
- Yelling
- Biting
- Hitting
- Turning head away
- Silence
- Echolalia (repetitive speech)
- Crying
- Pushing
- Rocking
- Wiggling
- Repetitive actions

What do these behaviors indicate?

IMPROBABLE		MORE LIKELY
- Willfulness		- Need to change activity
- Uncontrollable		- Visual stress
- Naughty	OR	- Boredom
- Uncooperative		- Fatigue
- Unmotivated		- Activity too easy
- Short attention span		- Activity too difficult

Other Behavior Signs to Monitor:

A change in:
- Posture
- Body tightness
- Speed
- Breathing
- Facial color

**When a person is handicapped in any visual task because of a visuo-motor problem, or when fatigue is building up because of excessive energy consumption related to visual work, behavior tends to deteriorate.
The child becomes nervous and more irritable.**

Relaxation

Purpose: Awareness and ability to keep the body in a relaxed state.

Teaching Deep Breathing

1. Breathe in through the nose - hold for a count of 4 - SLOWLY breathe out through the mouth - REPEAT for 5 to 10 minutes. Once you have learned this technique, incorporate deep breathing into your routine daily to encourage relaxation in stressful situations.

2. BLOW on hand: Blow on the hand of the child. Have them blow on their hand. The harder the blowing, the bigger the breath. REMEMBER to do this SLOWLY - VERY SLOW - BIG BREATH.

3. BLOW a feather: Move it so that it goes in the opposite direction

4. Hum and walk

5. Sing and walk

Deep breathing gets oxygen to the entire body and enhances relaxation.

Tight - Loose

Purpose: Teach the difference between a tight and relaxed body.

1. Have the child lie on the bed or on the floor on the stomach or the back.
   - Tighten the whole body, hold for 5 seconds, then relax the whole body
   - Tighten one arm (keep the rest of the body relaxed) then relax the arm.
   - Tighten any individual body part and relax

2. Stand tall, hold the arms above the head and tighten the whole body.
   - Bend at the waist, have the arms flop down and have the body relax.
   - Tighten, relax

Strenuous exercise forces deep breathing.

Writing

Discuss keeping the rest of the body relaxed while writing. Say in a soft, relaxed voice, "Take a deep breath and let's begin." He may even lose his temper and become erratic in his behavior.[8]

A relaxed body take less energy to move and direct.

Appendix A
Pre-Reading

Kathryn A. Koch,
Education Department,
University of Wisconsin, Green Bay, WI

All of these skills can be taught.

THINK of creative and unique ideas of reason for his/her ideas. Identifies the main idea and important details from stories.

UNDERSTANDS the relationship between words such as up/down, top/bottom, over/under and big/little.

REMEMBERS several directions and completes them in the correct order. Retells stories, songs and finger plays.

LISTENS to children and adults to directions without interrupting; to advice and constructive criticism without crying; to stories and poems for 10 to 15 minutes without restlessness.

HEARS words that rhyme; words that begin with the same sound.

SEES likenesses and differences in pictures, letters and words that match.

IDENTIFIES AND LABELS: letters of the alphabet; numbers from 0 - 10; basic shapes; colors

SPEAKS CLEARLY: and has a large oral vocabulary and stays on the topic during discussions.

KNOWS: how to print his/her first name basic information such as address, phone number, brothers, sisters, and birth date.

WORKS: without being easily distracted and completes each task and takes pride in his/her work and accepts and learns from mistakes.

PLAYS: cooperatively with other children and shares, takes turns, and assumes his/her share of group responsibility and can run, skip, jump, and bounce a ball.

ADJUSTS: to change in routine and to new situations without becoming fearful to the necessity of asking for help when needed to being away from home.

OBEYS: all teachers and school personnel class, playground, and school bus rules as established by the teacher.

Appendix B
Motor Skills

It doesn't matter where you are on the developmental scale. Teach what hasn't been learned automatically.

AGE 2: Walks well

Walks backward

Walks up steps

Knocks ball forward

Builds a tower of 3 - 4 blocks

Turns pages of a book looking at pictures naming or pointing to them

Thumb - finger grasp developed

Scribbles spontaneously

AGE 3: Throws ball overhand

Jumps in place

Pedals tricycle well

Broad jumps

Balances on one foot one second

Runs without falling

Squats in play

Performs rhythmical responses as bending knees in bouncing, swaying, swinging arms, nodding head, and tapping feet

Walks on tip toe

Jumps on 2 feet

Pushes toy with good steering

Runs, gallops and swings to music

Can carry a breakable object

Sees items and reaches almost simultaneously

Fits toys together

Locates picture in a picture book

Rotates forearm and turns down knob

Builds block horizontally or vertically in single line or tower

Attempts making vertical and horizontal lines, dots, and circular movements

Can turn pages of a book one at a time

AGE 4: Balances on one foot for five seconds
Walks erect and is confident in his movements
Can throw a ball without losing balance
Gallops, walks, runs, and jumps to music
Builds tower of eight cubes
Can copy a circle
Can put on shoes
Can unbutton layer buttons
Achieves order and balance in block building
May use non-dominant hand or shift handedness
Can turn sharp corners, dodge, stop and go
Can combine a vertical and horizontal crayon strokes to make a cross
Coordinates arms and legs well - left foot forward with right arm forward
Jumps and hops for 2 - 3 times

AGE 5: Hops on one foot 4 - 5 times
Walks heel to toe
Balances easily - can carry a full cup of liquid without spilling
Draws objects with few details
Uses scissors and attempts to cut a straight line
Laces shoes
Buttons front buttons
Catches a playground ball bounced chest high from a distance of 15 feet
Walks a 2" wide line without falling off for 10 - 15 feet

AGE 6: Balances on one foot for 10 seconds
Catches bounced ball
Walks backward heel-toe
Jumps from table height
Alternates feet descending stairs
Skips with alternate feet
Can march to music
Tries to roller skate, jump rope and to walk on stilts
Manipulates sand making roads and houses
Molds objects with clay
Likes to color within lines, to cut and paste simple things but is not always adept

Builds blocks generally on floor with towers or rambling structures with road and houses

Likes to copy simple forms

Can "sew" string through cards by turning over the cards

Laces shoes

Prints name correctly

Can hop rhythmically 10 - 15 feet

Walk a 4" wide balance beam (6" from ground) alternating feet without falling off

AGE 7: Skips to music

Bounces and tosses balls

Tries skating, running broad jump, and does stunts on bars

AGE 8: Galloping actions

Simple running step to music

Hops rhythmically from foot to foot in a 3 - 3 or 2 - 2 pattern

Executes a jumping jack smoothly

Walks a 2" wide balance beam 4 - 6" and 10 to 15' long without falling off

AGE 9: Body movements rhythmical and graceful

Learns soccer and baseball with softball

Runs into moving rope and can run out but not able to vary step while jumping

Standing position and movement free while painting

Writes or prints all letters and numbers accurately with fairly uniform slant, spacing and size

Throws a tennis ball over 50 feet

Shoots a basketball into a 8' - 10" high basket

Holds a one-foot balance with eyes closed

Holds a heel-toe position with arms folded across chest

Executes an alternating hopping pattern of 2 - 3 after it is demonstrated

Jumps rope rhythmically

Plays hop scotch

AGE 10: Interested in team games and learning to perform skillfully

Appendix C
Glossary
Children's Vision & The Learning Process

by Howard M. Coleman, O.D., M.Ed

There are certain visual-auditory-perceptual-motor constructs that are necessary for cognition, meaningful language, sensory processing and problem solving. Some of these are as follows:

Auditory Discrimination: Discrimination of pitch, loudness, speech sounds, and noises.

Auditory Figure-Ground: Selection of relevant form irrelevant auditory stimuli.

Auditory Sequential Memory: Discrimination and/or reproduction of patterns involving pitch, rhythm, and speech.

Figure-Ground: The discrimination of an object from its background.

Kinesthetic Discrimination: Perception derived from bodily movement including dynamic movement patterns, static limb positions, and sensitivity to direction.

Perceptual-Motor Discrimination: Both gross and fine motor skills are associated with all input systems. Bodily movement is necessary for locomotion and manipulation. Fine motor acts associated with visually expressive activity such as writing are often spoken of as visua-graphic. Much motor activity is involved in expressive auditory activity including speech, tongue movement, and jaw movement.

Spatial Relationships: The knowledge of one's body position in space and the perception of this position in relationship to other objects. Body-image acts as a zero locus or a point of reference in terms of knowledge of the individual's space world. Any fault in this body image will be reflected in the perception of outside objects.

Sound Awareness: Discrimination of sound vs. no sound.

Sound Localization: Awareness of source or direction of sound.

Tactile Perception: Perceptions of the environment including size, shape, texture, consistency, pain, and pressure.

Visual Closure: The identification of figures when only fragmentary clues are presented.

Visual-Discrimination: The discrimination of dominant features in different objects.

Visual Memory: Recognition of dominant features of one stimulus item or recalling the sequences of several items.

Children's Vision & The Learning Process

The following are terms utilized frequently in visual evaluations and are presented so that parents, educators, and other professionals will understand their meaning and not be caught up in a semantic jungle.

Accommodation: The process or mechanism of focusing the eye to enable a clear focus of near point material on the retina.

Astigmatism: That condition of the eye wherein the refracting surface and media are irregular and non-spherical causing more than one focus to fall upon the retina.

Binocular Vision: The resultant cortical integration of innervational patterns received from the eyes when they are both aligned on the target.

Brain-Eye-Hand Coordination: The ability to control the hand and eye movements of the body in coordination with visual-perceptual and visual-motor activity.

Convergence: The ability to turn the eyes inward bilaterally. Necessary in reading.

Depth Perception or Stereopsis: The ability to judge distance and the localization of the body in space.

Directionality: The projection of the internal concepts of laterality into external space.

Fixation: The ability to accurately control eye movement and direction to align on an object of regard.

Fusion: The cortical ability to interpret the stimuli received from simultaneous perception, and combine these stimuli into a total and single image of the object and regard.

Gestalt: Concepts of the form wherein an object is not perceived as component parts but rather as an entity of whole.

Hyperopia: That condition of the eye wherein the refractive power of the eye is less than "normal", and entering parallel rays of light come to a focus behind the retina.

Laterality: The internal awareness of the two sides of the body and their differences.

Muscle Balance: The study of the condition of the extra-ocular muscles to determine their degree of coordinated activity.

Myopia: That which is also known as nearsightedness. Condition of the eye wherein the refractive power is greater than "normal", and entering parallel rays of light come to a focus in front of the retina.

Ocular Motility: The ability of the extra-ocular muscles to move the eye through the various positions of gaze in response to stimuli.

Refractive Error: Any deviation from the normal visual state, correctable in general with spectacle or contact lenses.

Simultaneous Perception: That phenomenon wherein the cortical levels o f the occipital regions of the brain receive stimuli at the same time and at corresponding points.

Strabismus: That condition wherein the extra-ocular muscles are not in a state of balance, and a dysfunction of the fusion is present, resulting in eyes that are not in alignment. This misalignment can be up, down, in or out.

Visual Acuity: The ability to see an object clearly. If the object is blurred, the type and percentage of blur can be measured.

References

1. Seiderman AS, Marcus SE. 20/20 Is Not Enough. New York: Alfred A Knopf, 1990.

2. Hudson DL. Children Must Be Taught How To See. United International Publications, 1985.

3. Getman GN. How To Develop a Child's Intelligence. Santa Ana, CA: Optometric Extension Program Foundation, 1998.

4. Frostig M. Movement Education: Theory and Practice. Chicago: Follett Educational Corporation, 1970.

5. A Brighter Way of Life For All Children A Doctrine For Children. Developmental Care and Guidance, 1970.

6. Radler DH. Success Through Play. H. New York: Harper & Row, 1960.

7 Gesell A, Ilg FL, Bullis GE. Vision, its development in infant and child. Santa Ana, CA: Optometric Extension Program Foundation, 1998.

8. Blouin JP. The Black Book of the Year 2000. Santa Ana, CA: Optometric Extension Program Foundation, 19991.

9. Spache G, Hinds LR, Bing L. Vision and School Success. Santa Ana, CA: Optometric Extension Program Foundation, 1992.

Acknowledgments

Janet Chase, O.T.R, instructor of mental health in O.T.; private practice in psychiatric O.T., developmental disabilities; private consultant.

Howard Coleman, MEd, O.D., private optometric and therapy practice in Rumford, Rhode Island.

Joanne Kleist, executive director (assistant superintendent K-12 curriculum of instruction of the School District of Waukesha, Wisconsin).

John Muller, O.D., private optometric and therapy practice in Green Bay, Wisconsin.

Sharon Roberts, O.D., private optometric practice in Plymouth, Wisconsin, and therapy practice in Fond du Lac, Wisconsin

I'd like to thank my husband, Paul, for not ever letting me quit.

Thank you also to my children, Mickey, Tricia, Ben and Amy for weathering the up and downs of creating this book. I greatly appreciate Donna Wendelburg who opened a vocation to me and has never let me quit learning. Thanks to Mom and Dad for always believing in me, and teaching me every individual has value.

A special thank you to Marianne Taylor for carrying the torch for vision development long after her husband Fenwick's death.

Kathy Nurek

I am grateful for the teaching, support, encouragement and impetus of my teachers Howard Coleman, MEd, O.D., Ben Dander, O.D., John Muller, O.D., William Sorenson, O.D.

The goal is to use the knowledge to enrich the lives of all I meet.

Thanks to my parents who love unconditionally and give continually.

Thanks to my son, Jay, for being.

Thanks to Kathy Nurek for making the day to day progress possible and for keeping the dreams alive.

Donna Wendelburg